BONE MARROW
NEI KUNG

I have come upon Master Chia's Taoist practice in my old age and find it the
most satisfying and enriching practice of all those I have encountered in a
long life of seeking and practicing.

Felix Morrow,
Healing Tao Books

BONE MARROW NEI KUNG

Taoist Ways to Improve Your Health by Rejuvenating Your Bone Marrow and Blood

Mantak Chia
&
Maneewan Chia

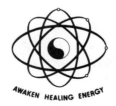

AWAKEN HEALING ENERGY

HEALING TAO BOOKS/Huntington, New York

BONE MARROW NEI KUNG
by Mantak and Maneewan Chia

DESIGN AND PRODUCTION: David Miller and Arlene Goldberg
EDITORS: Valerie Meszaros and Charles Soupios
PUBLISHING AND EDITING CONSULTANT: Joel Friedlander
EDITORIAL CONTRIBUTORS: Michael Winn, Dennis O'Connor, Eric Edelstein, Juan Li, Ron Diana
ILLUSTRATOR: Juan Li

First Published in 1989 by
Healing Tao Books
P.O. Box 1194
Huntington, NY 11743

Fifth Printing

ISBN: 0-935621-17-2
Library of Congress Card Number: 88-83169

Manufactured in the United States of America

10 9 8 7 6 5

Contents

3. The Sexual Energy Massage   87

The International Healing Tao System   Catalog 1-40

Important Notice

The practices described in this book have been done successfully for thousands of years by Taoists under individual instruction. Readers who undertake Bone Marrow Nei Kung without personal training by the Healing Tao must realize that certain of these practices, if improperly done, may cause injury or result in health problems.

The use of common sense is necessary, and you must strictly follow the instructions and heed the notices and warnings that accompany each exercise and practice.

If you have not had previous experience with moving energy in the body through meditation, you must realize that this process is real and necessary for your safety. Adverse health effects can be caused by leaving excess energy in the organs or head; therefore, it is particularly important to move this energy through the Microcosmic Orbit and to store it in the Tan Tien as prescribed in the instructions.

The Chi Weight Lifting practice described in Chapter Five is restricted to persons who have been individually trained in a Healing Tao program. It is explained here so that information on this practice is available, and also to serve as a guide for those who have had Healing Tao instruction. Anyone who undertakes these practices on the basis of this book does so entirely at his or her own risk.

We urge every reader to study the exercises carefully before beginning any practice. Do exercises which must be done together and in proper sequence, and strictly follow the instructions, notes, and warnings.

The Healing Tao is not and cannot be responsible for the consequences of any practice or misuse of the information in this book. Where the reader undertakes any exercise without strictly following the instructions, notes, and warnings, the responsibility must lie solely with the reader.

Acknowledgments

I wish to thank foremost those Taoist Masters who were kind enough to share their knowledge with me, never dreaming it would be so enthusiastically received by the Western world.

I thank the artist, Juan Li, for his illustrations and for the artwork on the cover of this book. I also thank the editors, Charles Soupios and Valerie Meszaros, for their suggestions and many long hours devoted to the completion of *Bone Marrow Nei Kung*.

Further, I wish to express my gratitude to the contributing editors, Michael Winn, Dennis O'Connor, Eric Edelstein, Juan Li, and particularly Ron Diana, all of whom contributed much to the technical aspects of this practice.

There were many other contributors who graciously offered their time and advice to help communicate this system, including Gunther Weil, Ph.D., Rylin Malone, and John-Robert Zielinski. Special thanks are extended to David Miller for overseeing the design and production, and to John Sillari and Marlene San Miguel Groner for proofreading the text.

Without my mother, my wife Maneewan, and my son Max, the book would have been academic. For their gifts, I offer my eternal gratitude and love.

Finally, the Healing Tao will remember Felix Morrow, publisher of Healing Tao Books, who died in May before the completion of *Bone Marrow Nei Kung*. We are sorry that he could not see the results of his valuable advice and assistance.

Words of Caution

When a person becomes aware of the poor condition of his or her health, the tendency is often to blame that which makes the problem known. Certainly one should consult a physician when in doubt about the benefits of any new approach to health. It would be wise, however, to look back to the roots of any problems that occur, rather than to the practice which reveals them. Any malady or condition which might be realized through Bone Marrow Nei Kung may not be the result of its practice. Consider also that the knowledge of impending danger to one's health is something for which one can be thankful.

Chinese medicine emphasizes balancing and strengthening the body so that it can heal itself. The meditations, internal exercises, and martial arts of the Healing Tao are basic approaches to this end. Follow the instructions for each exercise carefully, and do not neglect the supplemental exercises, particularly the Microcosmic Orbit Meditation. Also pay special attention to the warnings and suggestions in each chapter. People who have high blood pressure, heart disease, or a generally weak condition should proceed cautiously. Those with venereal disease should not attempt any practices involving sexual energy until they are free of the disease.

It is emphasized that the meditations described herein are NOT to be used as an alternative to professional medical treatment. This book does not give any diagnoses or suggestions for medication. If there are illnesses, especially mental problems, a medical doctor or psychologist should be consulted. Such problems should be corrected before you start training.

About Master Mantak Chia and Maneewan Chia

Master Chia

Master Mantak Chia is the creator of the Healing Tao system and the Director of the Healing Tao Center in New York. Since childhood he has been studying the Taoist approach to life as well as other approaches. His mastery of this ancient knowledge, enhanced by his study of other disciplines, has resulted in the development of the Healing Tao System which is now being taught in the United States, Canada, Europe, Australia, and Thailand.

Master Chia was born in Thailand to Chinese parents in 1944. When he was six years old, Buddhist monks taught him how to sit and "still the mind." While he was a grammar school student, he first learned traditional Thai boxing and then was taught Tai Chi Chuan by Master Lu, who soon introduced him to Aikido, Yoga, and more Tai Chi.

Later, when he was a student in Hong Kong excelling in track and field events, a senior classmate named Cheng Sue-Sue introduced him to his first esoteric teacher and Taoist Master, Master Yi Eng. At this point, he began his studies of the Taoist way of life. He learned how to circulate energy through the Microcosmic Orbit, how to open the Six Special Channels, Fusion of the Five Elements, Inner Alchemy, Enlightenment of the Kan and Li, Sealing of the Five Sense Organs, Congress of Heaven and Earth, and Reunion of Man and Heaven. He was soon able to clear blockages to the flow of energy within his own body. It was Master Yi Eng who authorized Master Chia to teach and heal.

In his early twenties Mantak Chia studied with Master Meugi in

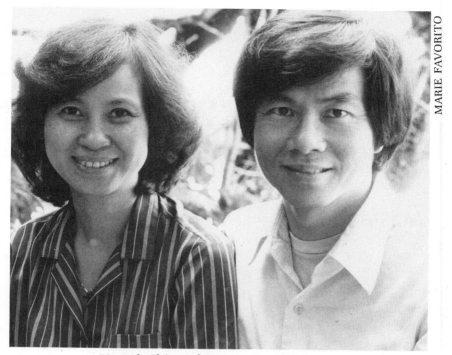

Mantak Chia and Maneewan Chia

Singapore, who taught him Kundalini, Taoist Yoga, and the Buddhist Palm. Master Meugi also taught him how to pass life-force energy through his hands to heal the patients of Master Meugi.

Later, he studied with Master Cheng Yao-Lun who taught him the Shao-Lin Method of Internal Power and the closely guarded secret of the organs, glands, and bone marrow exercise known as "Bone Marrow Nei Kung" and the "Strengthening and Renewal of the Tendons." Master Cheng Yao-Lun's system combined Thai boxing and Kung Fu. At this time he also studied with Master Pan Yu, whose system combined Taoist, Buddhist, and Zen teachings. From Master Pan Yu he learned about the exchange of the Yin and Yang power between men and women, and also how to develop the "Steel Body."

To better understand the mechanisms behind the healing energy, Master Chia studied Western medical science and anatomy for two years. While pursuing his studies, he managed the Gestetner Company, a manufacturer of office equipment, and became well-acquainted with the technology of offset printing and copying machines.

18

Using his knowledge of Taoism combined with the other disciplines, Master Chia began teaching the Healing Tao System. He eventually trained other teachers to communicate this knowledge, and he established the Natural Healing Center in Thailand. Five years later, he decided to move to New York where, in 1979, he opened the Healing Tao Center. Since then, centers have been opened in many other locations including Boston, Philadelphia, Denver, Seattle, San Francisco, Los Angeles, San Diego, Tucson, and Toronto. Groups are also forming in England, Germany, the Netherlands, Switzerland, Austria, and in Australia and Thailand.

Master Chia leads a peaceful life with his wife Maneewan, who teaches Taoist Five Element Nutrition at the New York Center, and their young son Max. He is a warm, friendly, and helpful man who views himself primarily as a teacher. He presents the Healing Tao in a simple, practical manner, always expanding his approach to teaching. He uses a word processor for writing, and is very much at ease with the latest in computer technology.

He has previously written and published six Healing Tao Books: in 1983, *Awaken Healing Energy through the Tao*; in 1984, *Taoist Secrets of Love: Cultivating Male Sexual Energy*; in 1985, *Taoist Ways to Transform Stress into Vitality*; in 1986, *Chi Self-Massage: The Tao Way of Rejuvenation*, *Iron Shirt Chi Kung I*, and *Healing Love through the Tao: Cultivating Female Sexual Energy*. *Bone Marrow Nei Kung* is his seventh book.

Maneewan Chia

Born and raised through her early years in Hong Kong, Maneewan Chia eventually moved with her parents to Thailand where she grew up to attend the University and earn a B.S. Degree in Medical Technology. Since childhood, Mrs. Chia has been very interested in nutrition and Chinese health food cooking. She learned by assisting her mother who was known as one of the finest cooks of her village. Since her marriage to Mantak Chia, she has studied the Healing Tao System and currently assists him in teaching classes and running the Healing Tao Center.

Introduction

Bone Marrow Nei Kung is a Taoist art of internal cultivation which employs mental and physical techniques to rejuvenate the bone marrow, thereby enhancing the blood and nourishing the life-force within. It is offered by the Healing Tao as a modern approach to health and longevity, but its heritage can be traced back thousands of years to ancient China. The barriers between cultures and the exclusivity of Taoism had hidden its benefits from the West until the recent introduction of acupuncture. Today, Taoist methods are gaining respect throughout the world. The reason for this is simple: they appeal to the body, the mind, and the spirit.

The Healing Tao system is a "living" philosophy in its own right, which means that to use it in life increases one's understanding of it. Indeed, with so many philosophies delineating the "best" way to live, perhaps it is appropriate that the Taoist practices can be applied in this way. A philosophy that cannot be practiced in daily life will rarely be retained, and is therefore not truly alive. If you consider your own mental, physical and spiritual aspirations in this light, perhaps the philosophy of the Tao is already understood.

A. SELF-ENHANCEMENT THROUGH TAOIST PRACTICES

One objective of the Healing Tao System is to create an environment conducive to self-cultivation. The idea of changing a government, a belief system, or a society has little value to Taoism because more can be achieved by nurturing the growth of the individual. Those who seek knowledge often inspire others to do the same. This may seem strange to those whose philosophies advocate service to God, or "self-surrender." The validity of this concept, however, is not diminished simply because its ideals seem contrary. In fact, one might find that self-cultivation and self-surrender are different expressions of the same ideal as both foster the individual's spiritual growth.

The practice of Taoism builds internal strength and creates peace of mind. It is pointless to worry about the world's problems while still vulnerable to your own. Do not concern yourself with the lack of peace and harmony in your family or among your friends until you have established peace within yourself. Your capacity to help another human being depends upon the surplus of energy that you can channel towards that purpose. Such internal strength cannot be provided for the benefit of others unless you cultivate it within yourself first.

You can only share what you have in abundance. Otherwise, you will drain the energies of those around you as your needs become excessive. An emotion such as love exemplifies this truth. Taoism teaches that the body needs love from the inner self to survive and to nurture those energies that can be shared. Further, you cannot share the energy of love until it overflows beyond the needs of your body. In other words, you must love yourself to cultivate love for others.

In a spirit of altruism, people often demonstrate their desire to assist others beyond the point of necessity. This kind of "help" is detrimental to all concerned. Remember that the tradition of the Healing Tao does not tolerate self-righteousness and condescension among its students. These attitudes limit the freedom of others to choose their own paths in life. The world must be accepted on its own terms, for we cannot change it. We have a responsibility, however, to change ourselves. If you can set an example for the rest of the world through your life's endeavors, then you have found the best way to create an impetus for change.

B. DECISIONS FOR LIFE

We assume that it is natural to age and to die, yet we often overlook the unnatural aspects of these processes by anticipating them. In truth, today's society simply lacks the education to understand how aging and death are choices we have made in our worldly endeavors. This is not to say that the human race is unknowingly immortal, but rather that we have far more control over these factors than we know. Death can be a choice in the sense that we can choose to live longer. Aging is a choice in that our bodies need not deteriorate as an effect of time. The effects of aging can be counteracted if we make the choice to do so. Certainly we all die, but we have forgotten that we all have options as to how and when.

Taoists choose to prolong life to create the best circumstances under which they can leave it. Since people know little about realities beyond physical existence, they often fear such knowledge, leaving it in the hands of God. This is how our race has learned survival under the most rigorous conditions of faith. However, this fear has often negated the inner knowledge that God is not responsible for mankind's spiritual search; man is responsible. In Taoism, destiny lies solely in the hands of the participant and not in the hands of God, for we choose our actions in life.

The Taoist practice of temporarily leaving the body to explore the higher realms is as old as the most ancient of civilizations. This need not involve any confrontation with religion. It is part of a philosophy of life using physical and meditative means to cultivate spiritual energy. In the practice of the Healing Tao, this philosophy is not considered to be a religion because it lacks the rituals and worship of deities normally associated with religion. Consider, however, that religion is not necessarily synonymous with spirituality, since our true spiritual nature underlies the beliefs we grow into. Taoist philosophy simply offers a means of spiritual growth without the necessity of pondering religious questions. In the search for truth, one can leave the questions in order to experience the answers.

For some people, the idea of planning to journey beyond what can be physically touched or seen is totally inappropriate. This is perfectly reasonable in terms of spiritual growth because there is much to be learned in the world that we know. There is no reason for anyone to suffer in this reality, when good health can be achieved through these techniques. If one so chooses, one can develop the beginning of a spiritual afterlife before physical death would normally occur. For those who prefer to cultivate only the physical aspects of life, the copious health benefits of the Tao should be rewarding enough. The choice is simple in any case as the system is now available to everyone.

Remember that there is no place in Taoism for the glorification of masters. They are not saints, devils, or deities. These teachers consider it a wasteful expenditure of energy for students to pay them anything more than a casual, but genuine, respect. Taoist philosophy suggests that no "middle-man" is worth the expense when we can find our own answers. The enlightenment we seek demands that our efforts be channeled directly into the spiritual paths we choose. Those who would teach should only be considered helpful guides who offer assistance rather than salvation.

There are many more disciplines available than we need to attain enlightenment. Our spiritual inclinations, therefore, must eventually focus upon choosing wisely rather than searching endlessly. A Taoist cannot rely upon the good graces of a spiritual hierarchy because it is one's own responsibility to learn what spiritual needs are and how to fulfill them. The physical life we have chosen has many tools to offer. The Tao is simply a finger pointing the way.

Preface

CHINESE SECRETS OF BONE POWER

by Michael Winn

When I began doing Bone Marrow Nei Kung exercises seven years ago, I had absolutely no feeling for my bones. They seemed hard, rigid, and dense, the very opposite of the qualities I was seeking to cultivate in myself through Tai Chi Chuan movements and meditation. I didn't know my bones were alive and growing every minute, that my life depended on the quality of blood they produced, or that I could have a major effect on my health by interacting with them.

I was amazed and surprised that with even the simplest exercises like "Bone Breathing," my bones quickly responded with a wonderful feeling of just having sprung to life. They tingled and began to rhythmically purr like a cat. When I did Tai Chi Chuan, my flesh and organs would disappear, and I could feel my skeleton dancing lightly through the air.

Over the years, doing the same simple practice of breathing and spiraling my Chi around my bones, I am still literally "thrilled to the bone." After I practice "Hitting" my bones gently, it feels like a deep massage that keeps vibrating all day long. The practices have greatly reduced latent fears I had of aging and finding my bones reduced to peanut brittle. Instead, I have the opposite problem, and I'm tickled when my wife complains that my bones have gotten too heavy as she tosses off my arm resting on her in the middle of the night.

Any lingering skepticism I had was erased when I discovered that hitting my jawbone with the wire device for three minutes daily was the most effective cure I had ever found for relieving tight jaw muscles. Jaws have some of the most powerful muscles in the body, which is why TMJ (Temporal Mandibular Joint) Syndrome (a symptom of which is tight jaw muscles) is so difficult to cure. Apparently vibrating the jawbone loosens the hold of the tense muscles. This method offers promising relief for the many people suffering from tight jaw muscles in high stress urban areas.

My bones and I have become the best of friends now that I've learned how to play with them and meditate on them. Bone Marrow Nei Kung has given me a practical way to connect the densest part of my physical body with the most subtle emanations of my spirit. The meaning of a Yang family classic Tai Chi Chuan training poem suddenly became clear once I understood the importance of moving from within our bones:

> The mind moves the Chi
> So that it may sink deeply and penetrate the bones
> When the Chi flows freely,
> The body easily follows the mind

"Cleansing" my bone marrow was not always smooth sailing. In the beginning, the process of heavy detoxification was not always pleasant, and I occasionally felt ill for a day or two. There were psychological adjustments as well. Exercises like "Chi Weight Lifting" with the sexual organs and the Hitting practice seemed a bit far out at first. I cracked a lot of nervous jokes about religious fanatics flagellating themselves with whips, and I secretly wondered if I had fallen prey to some extreme teaching.

Having practiced these exercises for almost seven years now, I can assure the reader that the Bone Marrow Nei Kung practices are legitimate exercises for physical and spiritual health. The ancient Chinese were incredibly precise, even scientific in their methods of tapping bone power. Mantak Chia has taken this one step further by integrating modern scientific knowledge of bone chemistry with the ancient knowledge of Chi functioning in the human bones and body.

The name "Bone Marrow Nei Kung" sounds pretty mysterious and esoteric. Master Chia originally taught it as an advanced level of "Iron Shirt Chi Kung." It may help to understand the cultural context of these Chinese terms. In China there are thousands of different "Chi Kung" practices taught by martial artists and meditation masters. Chi Kung literally means "practicing with the breath," which can include any exercise that uses breathing to energize the body. The physical breath activates the "Chi," also interpreted as "subtle breath," which generates increased physical and psychic strength.

Chi Kung is still so popular that on a recent trip to China I saw hundreds of Chinese flock to circus-like traveling road shows that gave Chi Kung top billing. These Chi Kung artists, with no apparent muscular buildup, perform feats like bending thick steel rods pushed into the soft spot on their necks. They break bricks on their heads, let trucks drive over them, and resist sharp knives with their bare skin.

These are high levels of physical accomplishment, but unfortunately they miss the real point of Chi Kung, which is to prepare the body for higher spiritual energies. Through Kung Fu movies and Chi Kung showmen, the practice of Chi Kung has been glorified as a path to superhuman physical power. This frightens off ordinary people from learning the true practices which are simple and give great benefits to health.

"Nei Kung" is a very close relative to Chi Kung. It means "practicing with your internal power" and implies building body-mind power without using physical breathing techniques. Mental concentration, internal imaging, and development of a deep inner sensing of psychophysical processes are the marks of Nei Kung techniques.

Most of the methods of internal alchemy taught at the Healing Tao centers—the Inner Smile, Microcosmic Orbit, Fusion of the Five Elements, Kan and Li—are all "Nei Kung" techniques. Perhaps because they are more subtle than Chi Kung methods, the Nei Kung methods are fewer in number, and traditionally many have been kept very secret.

When Master Chia visited Taiwan in 1987, he discovered that the going price to learn Bone Marrow Nei Kung was about four thousand U.S. dollars for ten hours of instruction. Plus you had to take an oath of absolute secrecy not to teach anyone else. Master Chia had already learned the practice in Hong Kong more than a decade earlier from Master Cheng Yao-Lun.

When Master Chia learned the method of "Cleansing the Bone Marrow," the price was years of slavish devotion until your teacher, or "Sifu," entrusted you with the secrets. When he completed his training, it was Chia's very impatience with this slow process that inspired him to publish these closely guarded secrets to benefit the thousands of Westerners seeking accurate and practical instruction in Chinese internal arts.

The previously secret Bone Marrow Nei Kung methods of this book are the same ones associated with stories of masters achieving an "iron shirt" or building a "steel body." Contrary to movie legend, this is not a superman body of hardened flesh and muscle, but the inner strength of a body whose bones and organs are so packed with Chi energy that it resists aging and disease. The resilience to withstand the physical stress of hard blows or sudden falls comes from packing the fasciae with Chi that helps the body to "bounce off" outside forces.

Bone Marrow Nei Kung does generate tremendous amounts of Chi, and this makes it a dangerous practice for overzealous students who lack the self discipline to refine this Chi through meditation. The body can overheat from excess energy, and meditation is the safety valve that transforms this raw energy back into its original spirit or "shen."

This is why in the Healing Tao System it is necessary to learn the Microcosmic Orbit Meditation before one even begins generating additional energy through Chi Kung. Without some way to refine and use the energy, what is the point of cultivating internal power?

I know one advanced student who eagerly did the Chi Weight Lifting exercises of Bone Marrow Nei Kung to generate more sexual energy. He then vibrated it into his bones with the device used in the Hitting practice. He was lifting very heavy weights from his genitals, far in excess of the ten pounds recommended in this book. He was so addicted to his practice that he would carry a suitcase full of weights with him wherever he travelled.

The student made the serious mistake of not meditating to assimilate all of the energy he was creating. He began having dreams that various creatures and people were feeding on him, and he started to become very paranoid. He finally quit the practice altogether after a psychic told him that many low level spirits were parasitically absorbing his excess sexual energy. He quit lifting excessive weights and his energy returned to normal. This is a bizarre and somewhat incredible story, but it should serve as a warning to people who tend to go overboard on a new thing.

Even masters are not exempt from the dangers of over-zealousness. The Taiwanese teacher who was selling the Chi Weight Lifting techniques for thousands of dollars claimed to be able to briefly lift 300 pounds from his genitals. It proved to be too much for him as he recently died at a very young age, allegedly from a blood clot in his testicles that may have travelled up to his brain. Had he chosen to be more practical, using light weights in a regimen balanced with meditation, he might still be alive today.

In ancient China the Taoists who practiced internal cultivation of Chi saw a deep "bone consciousness" as an essential step on their long journey to realizing their immortality. According to the classic Taoist texts, when the postnatal Chi—all the energy acquired by food, sex, thoughts, and emotions since birth—circulates in the Microcosmic Orbit, it stirs loose the prenatal Chi stored in the bone marrow and the brain.

It is this prenatal Chi, also called pre-heaven or primordial Chi, that is refined into spiritual consciousness and gives birth to the immortal embryo in the lower abdomen. This grows up to become the spiritual child and eventually crystallizes into the "light body" or "immortal body" of the spiritually mature human.

For the Taoists, the bones were a secret key to stabilizing or "grounding" the life of the spirit within the human body. Before this could be done, the bones had to be cleansed, and their vibratory rate—bone consciousness—had to be raised to a more refined level. The movement of Chi in the bones was used to amplify the process of cleansing and purifying the Chi flowing through the meridian system, blood, internal organs, glands, and nervous system.

The bones create the vertical structure in man which allows special energy channels to function in the body such as the "Chung-mo," which is the thrusting route in the center of the body, and the "belt routes" spiraling around the body. These channels allow man to act as an antenna and receive energy from the electromagnetic fields of the earth, moon, sun, and stars—the stepping stones to our sense of divinity.

In this light, an entire book on Bone Marrow Nei Kung does not seem like such an impossibly esoteric topic. A few years ago this topic would have drawn interest from only select circles of martial artists. Yet Bone Marrow Nei Kung practices can be done by ordinary people who simply wish to be more embodied, more grounded, and healthier in their physical being. These practices were once extremely secret in old China, but today the secrets of the Tao are opening like a flower, and the sweet fragrance is available to anyone drawn to it.

Modern popular literature on bone health is limited mostly to diet and mineral supplement advice on preventing osteoporosis. This disease, which makes bones brittle with age as they become depleted of calcium, is a major tragedy for the elderly, especially women after menopause. Recent studies show that calcium supplements are of dubious value in stopping osteoporosis.

According to scientific studies, what does reverse the process of osteoporosis are exercises that put gentle pressure on the bones and keep them fit, combined with the proper hormonal balance in the body. Bone Marrow Nei Kung gives the bones exercise, increases bone density, and the Sexual Energy Massage technique helps to stimulate hormonal production. Millions of women would benefit from these exercises as a preventative measure against osteoporosis.

One exception to the gap in modern literature on bones is Gabriel Cousen's landmark book, Spiritual Nutrition and the Rainbow Diet (Cassandra Press, 1986). He points out that our bones are the only solid crystalline substance in our bodies and that scientists have actually been able to measure the electromagnetic fields that bones receive and send to our organs, meridians, blood cells, and nerves. The electrical generating ability of bones is called the "piezo-electric effect," and has been documented by a number of scientific studies. He states:

"The brain, nervous system, and heart also give off electromagnetic fields that resonate with our bones and other crystalline like structures. The crystalline bone structure then amplifies and radiates this energy and information to the rest of the system down to the cellular and subcellular crystalline structures."

This suggests the bones are nothing less than the tuning fork for our whole body. It is the solidity of the bones that makes them such stable transmitters of the deep, rhythmic, pulsating energy that biologically connects our smallest atoms to the primordial rhythms of the stars. Bone Marrow Nei Kung gives us a way to systematically increase the purity and range of our body's tuning fork so it hums with a crystal clear vibration.

Bone consciousness has manifested in a variety of other interesting ways outside of the martial arts. In the mainstream Chinese culture a deep reverence for bones is revealed in the great importance placed on burial and ancestor worship. If the bones of your parents or grandparents are buried near a disturbing environment with noise and traffic, or in a site with the wrong elemental balance of water, wind, mountain, etc., then your own life will be disturbed.

According to Chinese theory, this "bone magic" works because the vibrational frequency of your body is very close to the vibrational frequencies of your parents' bodies. If their bones are disturbed, your bones will also be disturbed as we always remain in subtle communication with those closest to ourselves. Our bones never die. They continue acting as transmitters for the departed spirit.

Our bones are like invisible wands concealed within the shrouds of our flesh. We wave them about in life like an orchestra conductor invoking the magic of the higher harmonies. It is when we get old that our bones feel empty and brittle, without the sparkle and dash needed to play life's symphony. And small wonder since we pound them, run and joggle them, use and abuse them in a thousand ways without even giving a thought to making them stronger. Gravity adds its stress by pulling down on them without allowing any relief.

Bone Marrow Nei Kung offers an opportunity to explore the core of our physical body and to learn how to root our spiritual being within that solid physical anchor. The benefits are universal, teaching us to use the unconscious power deep within our bones and make it available for mundane everyday use, as well as for spiritual goals.

The next step is up to us. We must experiment with the Bone Marrow Nei Kung exercises until we feel this ancient knowledge of Chi as a living presence in our bones. As Mantak Chia is fond of saying, "You do it, you get it."

New York City, July 4, 1988

Michael Winn is a senior instructor at the Healing Tao Center, and co-author, with Mantak Chia, of *Taoist Secrets of Love: Cultivating Male Sexual Energy.* A writer, photographer, and entrepreneur, he lives in New York with his wife and co-teacher, Anna Joy Gayheart.

Chapter One

UNDERSTANDING BONE MARROW NEI KUNG

A. INTERNAL DISCIPLINE VS. EXTERNAL EXERCISE

The Western world generally believes that daily physical exercise helps to slow the aging process. In our society physical fitness is gauged according to the external manifestations of arduous training. An example of this is the trend towards muscular development through weight lifting. Athletic competition has also influenced many of our concepts of health and well-being. If one considers, however, that body builders and athletes enjoy the same life span as the average human, one might reconsider the assumption that they are the most "physically fit."

The professional athletes we admire expend enormous amounts of energy to attain top positions in their sports. As they overdraw on their resources for long periods of time, their internal organs often lose the capability to feed such exhaustive energy requirements. The inexorable effects of aging then impede them until they can no longer compete. Some may delay the exhaustion of their energy sources through vitamins and nutrition, but their digestive capabilities usually decrease with age, making a dependency upon food and vitamins even less promising. Nutrition and physical exercise are not comprehensive approaches to health, even when they are combined.

In your own fitness training, you may be indirectly exercising the internal organs and glands; however, if you do not emphasize their cultivation above and beyond that of the muscular system, you can ultimately do more damage than good. The organs and glands nourish every function of the body, just as the bone marrow nourishes them through the production of blood. Still, we unknowingly tax the internal system beyond its limits because we believe that muscular development should take precedence. Without the energy supplied by the internal organs and glands, there can be no lasting muscular development. In short, muscular strength and stamina may not be the best medium by which to judge overall physical health.

The Taoist approach to health is very different from Western concepts of exercise because the Taoist disciplines are always internally focused. These exercises, therefore, emphasize the cultivation of the organs and glands. After the organs and glands have been enhanced, the needs of the tendons, bones, and muscles are fulfilled accordingly. Bone Marrow Nei Kung replenishes the blood supply and strengthens the internal system, thereby improving every aspect of the body.

Energizing the bone marrow is crucial to the development of that internal power which has a lasting quality unknown to external systems of health. We have all heard that inner beauty lasts when outer beauty begins to fade. The Taoist practices cultivate inner strength and lasting beauty, as they enhance the external aspects of the body.

B. BONE MARROW NEI KUNG AND THE PRACTICE OF THE HEALING TAO

1. The Internal Energy Known as Chi

Taoists describe the world as an interaction of positively and negatively charged electromagnetic energies. "Chi" is an overall term used for these energies, which comprise the ultimate nourishment derived from food, air, moon, sun, and stars. Chi is also generated within our bodies by the organs and glands, and it extends around us as part of our emanation. This is why the cultivation of our organs and glands is so important to the enhancement of our life-force energies.

Just as the positive and negative terminals of a battery must both be engaged to generate power in an electrical circuit, the "Yin" and "Yang" qualities of Chi must both be engaged for the proper functioning of the body. Yin is analogous to the negative charge, and represents a cool, gentle energy often associated with femininity. Yang is the positive charge, and represents a hot, volatile energy that is characteristic of masculinity. Both qualities can be found within us, although there is often a lack of harmony between them. The knowledge of Yin and Yang and their proper balance is critical to our daily lives because an imbalance can create a negative effect.

Chi—also known as "Qi"—is a constant factor in every part of our lives. Unfortunately, we often lose it at a faster rate than we can amass it. As our internal sources of energy are not inexhaustible, we can unknowingly drain them beyond repair, creating the possibility of painful aging and an early demise. If the organs and glands could regenerate themselves, however, such possibilities would become remote. Fortunately, what we have sacrificed of our bodies in our worldly pursuits can often be replaced through the absorption and recycling of Chi. In other words, this energy can be used to replenish its sources within our bodies so that we can regenerate our internal systems and better maintain them.

Chi cultivation is the underlying purpose of the Healing Tao. This is the essence of all that a practitioner of this system aspires to. If one wishes to be a healer, success depends upon the ability to channel energy through the hands. If one wishes to be an athlete, success depends upon the ability to convert energy into strength and endurance. If one wishes to be free of negative influences, success depends upon the ability to transform negative energy into positive energy. One who seeks enlightenment is searching for the highest source of all energy.

2. Bone Marrow Nei Kung in Theory

The purpose of Bone Marrow Nei Kung is to regenerate the blood-producing red marrow of the bones to enhance the blood and the sources of Chi within the body. The system consists of five practices related to the following functions:

a. Breathing in energy from external sources
b. Drawing in and circulating sexual energy throughout the body
c. Vibrating the bones to open their pores for energy absorption
d. Compressing the combined energies into the bones to
   eliminate fat
e. Enhancing the nervous and lymphatic systems while
   detoxifying the skin

The techniques of Bone Marrow Nei Kung reverse the effects of aging by regenerating the bone marrow with sexual energy while eliminating the accumulated fat which restricts the production of blood. Exercises are also used to detoxify the body and improve the functions of the nervous and lymphatic systems. Finally, a sixth practice is used by advanced practitioners to further strengthen the internal organs and glands by exercising the fascial layers which surround them. A higher concentration of sexual energy—referred to as Ching Chi—is released into the body through this technique.

Men have reported increased strength, endurance, and sexual powers upon mastering Bone Marrow Nei Kung. Women have reported that the Hitting techniques, used in conjunction with other exercises, are a perfect weapon against cellulite. Bone Marrow Nei Kung is also an excellent medium for weight control as it generates intense heat within the body to burn up large quantities of fat. This system can be used to enhance one's capabilities in all activities, including martial arts, running, weight lifting, football, aerobics, dance, and so on.

The exercises of Bone Marrow Nei Kung should not be considered a strict regimen. Progress is not contingent upon arduous practice except in a martial arts context where the goals are different. Those who cannot devote much time to esoteric disciplines should still be able to progress slowly but steadily to better health. Upon developing a reasonable proficiency with these techniques, practice can be curtailed to every other day, if necessary, to maintain that level of proficiency. These exercises and their prerequisites should only take from 35 minutes to one hour to complete.

C. AN OVERVIEW OF BONE MARROW NEI KUNG AND RELATED DISCIPLINES

1. The Practices of Bone Marrow Nei Kung

Bone Marrow Nei Kung—sometimes referred to as Iron Shirt Chi Kung III—consists of the five interrelated practices. Chi Weight Lifting is a sixth technique described in Chapter Five for advanced practitioners. With the exception of Chi Weight Lifting, all of the following exercises, including the supplemental practices, should be used in your training schedule to some extent. If you wish to receive instruction in these disciplines, it is advised that you contact the Healing Tao for information on the seminars in which Bone Marrow Nei Kung is taught.

a. The Bone Breathing Process: Bone Breathing uses the power of the mind with deep, relaxed inhalations to establish an inward flow of external energy through the fingertips and toes. This energy is used to complement previously stored sexual energy which is released into the body through the Sexual Energy Massage or Chi Weight Lifting and then compressed into the bones. The external energy helps to eliminate the fat accumulated in the bone marrow, thereby assisting in the marrow's regeneration. Bone Breathing may be used with or without Bone Compression, but they are presented as a combined practice in this book.

b. Bone Compression: After external energy has been breathed into a particular area, the muscle contractions of this process force the combined energies into the bones to burn the fat out of the marrow. While Bone Breathing is a mental process used in conjunction with long, soft breath cycles, Bone Compression is a physical process of contracting the muscles, thereby squeezing Chi into the bones. Combining the mental with the physical in this way enhances the results of Bone Marrow Nei Kung.

c. The purpose of the Sexual Energy Massage is to release Ching Chi from the genitals so that it can be disseminated throughout the body and absorbed into the bones. (The term "Ching Chi" actually refers to sexual energy and sexual hormones combined.) The fingers massage the genitals while meditative breathing is used to draw the sexual energy and hormones upward from the genitals into the body. The genitals are later replenished by the rejuvenated organs and the return flow of the Microcosmic Orbit Meditation, described in Chapter Six.

Although the combined energies from sexual and external sources are used to burn fat out of the bones, only Ching Chi can regenerate bone marrow. The massage techniques release tremendous amounts of Ching Chi into the body for this purpose. The release of sexual hormones into the bloodstream also stimulates the pineal and pituitary glands. Western science believes that the pituitary gland produces an aging hormone in the absence of this stimulation, contributing to an early death.

d. The first Hitting technique has two applications: one uses a form of compression to force Chi into the bones; the other works without any muscle tension. "Hitting with Packing" amplifies the Bone Compression practice, using a special device to strike each successive area of the body or limbs that is being compressed. The device creates vibrations throughout the body which open the pores of the bones to receive condensed energy. Specific lines correlating with known acupuncture meridians are hit along their respective lengths to open their channels for the energy flow.

In the second application, "Hitting to Detoxify," the striking device is applied without any form of Bone Compression, and the muscles stay relaxed. This detoxifies the body, helping it to absorb Chi. Hitting to Detoxify is recommended for beginning students because it has a less overwhelming effect on the body than the packing method. In both applications, Hitting is one of the most efficient techniques available for detoxifying the body.

e. The last technique, "Hitting with Rattan Sticks," employs a similar striking sequence to stimulate the nervous and lymphatic systems. The sticks do not emphasize vibrations as the wire device does, but the shock of their contact strengthens skin, muscles, tendons, and bones. (They should not be applied to the bones directly.) This method also detoxifies the skin, thereby improving the complexion. Hitting with Rattan Sticks completes the basic procedures of Bone Marrow Nei Kung.

f. Chi Weight Lifting is the last practice described in this text because of its advanced nature and its dependence on the other disciplines. It is similar to the Sexual Energy Massage, but weights are used to increase the pressure on the genitals. The procedure should not be attempted until all of the massage techniques in Chapter Three have been thoroughly mastered. Chi Weight Lifting differs from the Sexual Energy Massage in that it develops strength in the layers of fasciae surrounding the organs and glands. These tissues are engaged to counteract the downward pull of the weight against the genitals, thereby creating an upward flow of energy from the sexual center.

NOTE: Chi Weight Lifting is included herein to document its practice for instructors and trained students. It is not recommended for beginners or casual readers without a full understanding of its applications as taught at Healing Tao seminars.

g. Using the Bone Marrow Nei Kung Practices:

(1) Practitioners usually begin with Bone Breathing and Bone Compression to draw external energies into the body. (In advanced practice, you may prefer to use these steps only during the Hitting with Packing process.)

(2) Either the Sexual Energy Massage or Chi Weight Lifting techniques are then used to release Ching Chi, which is combined with the external energies.

(3) Finally, the Hitting practices must follow the release of sexual energy: First the vibrations are created to help the body assimilate the combined energies into the bones. Then the rattan sticks are used to strengthen the skin and nerves.

2. Required Supplemental Practices for Bone Marrow Nei Kung

The Healing Tao employs many other disciplines integral to Bone Marrow Nei Kung. Most of these practices can be used alone; however, a working knowledge of them all, including certain meditations, is necessary for Bone Marrow Nei Kung. It is the working knowledge of these other disciplines that creates a safer practice. After learning the required supplements, you may emphasize particular aspects of your training according to the needs of your body.

Tremendous energy is released during practice, which can cause an imbalance if one does not know how or where to channel and store an overflow of Chi. This could create problems that would require an acupuncturist to correct in order to avoid dangerous side effects. As a rule, hot energy is never allowed to remain in the organs and glands because it can overheat them. The supplemental practices used with Bone Marrow Nei Kung remove such an overflow of energy to the proper storage areas.

a. THE MICROCOSMIC ORBIT AND THE INNER SMILE

A common denominator of all the physical disciplines, as well as the mental and spiritual work, is the Microcosmic Orbit Meditation, which is initiated by the "Inner Smile." (See Chapter Six.) In relation to Bone Marrow Nei Kung, the flow of the Microcosmic Orbit is necessary for channeling sexual energy. (Figure 1-1) Ching Chi is drawn up from the lower centers into this flow and distributed throughout the body. In this way, meditation assists in creating blood cells by circulating Chi to enhance bone marrow.

WARNING: To practice without the Microcosmic Orbit Meditation can cause irregular heartbeat, chest congestion, headaches, pain in the chest or back, and other problems. This meditation is a prerequisite for Bone Marrow Nei Kung. IGNORE IT AT YOUR OWN PERIL.

b. HEALING LOVE

Another important exercise for Bone Marrow Nei Kung is the Healing Love practice used in all sexual activities. The loss of sexual energy, or "Ching Chi," depletes the bone marrow and the vital organs which must replace what was lost. Unless one learns how to retain this energy and build up a healthy reserve, the organs and glands must sacrifice one third of their energy to replenish the genitals which produce Ching Chi.

The Healing Love methods for both men and women involve drawing in orgasmic energy and channeling it upward to higher centers, thereby reversing the outward flow of Ching Chi that is normally released during sex. When used in conjunction with the Sexual Energy Massage, these techniques combine to release tremendous amounts

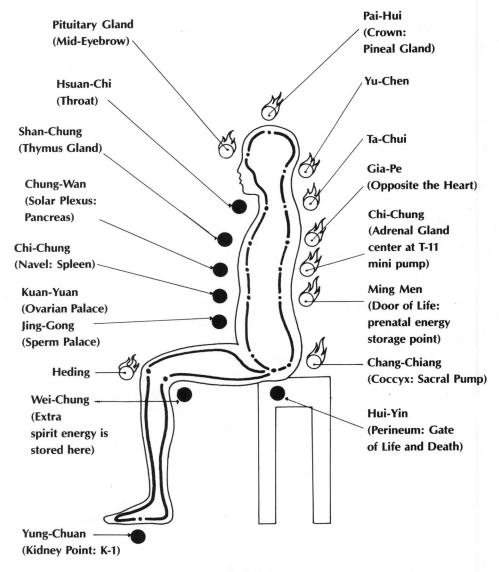

FIGURE 1-1

The Stations of the Microcosmic Orbit

of Ching Chi upward into the body, making this practice very useful to Bone Marrow Nei Kung. When used alone, Healing Love methods release abundant sexual energy which can then be stored and cultivated for mental, physical, and spiritual use.

Sexual energy can be transformed into life-force energy, compounded regularly by the Healing Love practice. The use of these methods not only improves the internal organs and glands but also enhances one's sexual satisfaction. The libido lasts for many more hours during sex, and for many more years in one's life. Furthermore, sexual stimulation reaches far beyond the conventional idea of a "climax."

c. IRON SHIRT CHI KUNG I

The postures of Iron Shirt I can be an excellent medium for the practice of Bone Marrow Nei Kung. In the Iron Shirt techniques, one learns to compress energy into the fasciae surrounding the organs and glands. These protective sheaths of tissue are most conducive to the Chi flow that nourishes the internal system.

Compression of Chi creates its storage space within the fasciae as the fat lodged within the muscles, tendons, and bones is purged and then transformed into more energy. A brief synopsis of the related postures is included in Appendix 1. Iron Shirt Chi Kung I is detailed in the Healing Tao book of the same name.

d. THE SIX HEALING SOUNDS

The Six Healing Sounds are produced sub-vocally and correspond to specific organs: the lungs, kidneys, liver, heart, and spleen. The sixth sound is the "Triple Warmer" which evenly distributes energy throughout the body. When used independently of Bone Marrow Nei Kung, each sound creates its own energy to enhance and detoxify the internal system. All six sounds and their related postures decelerate the body after practice and remove excess heat accumulated in vital areas. These exercises are fully explained in Appendix 1 and also in the Healing Tao book, *Taoist Ways to Transform Stress into Vitality*.

D. The Importance of Internal Exercises

The Master of Internal Strength

There once was a master who was very powerful. Many people wanted to learn from him, but he was difficult to have an audience with. This master felt that, unless one had patience, no one was worthy of his lessons. There was a very determined man, however, who waited three years, day after day, to see him. But the master would only appear to discourage those who waited. He would send them away, and they would all leave, except for this one man. Finally, the master became curious about this man who remained each day only to receive such disappointment.

One day the master asked the man, "If I tell you to do something, will you do it?" "I will try my best," the man answered. So the master told him to go over to a tree that grew nearby and pull it out of the ground for him. The man looked at the tree and decided to try it, since this was better than waiting for the treatment that the other people would get. He went over to the tree, grabbed it, and pulled at it. He did this day after day, year after year.

With each passing year, the tree grew bigger, but with each passing year, the man developed more internal strength. Finally one day, after ten years of daily effort, he became very determined to pull that tree out. He felt his body fill with Chi as he approached the tree and grabbed it. His feet were firmly planted on the ground, and he was wrapped around the tree in such a way that his internal strength could best be applied. With great force, he finally pulled the tree out.

The man went to the master and excitedly reported his great triumph. The master said that was fine, and then told him to leave. The man was very surprised and disturbed by the master's response. It appeared that he had been shunned without ever learning from this master after all. The master looked at him and said, "If you can pull that tree out of the ground, whoever in the world would want to fight you?" The man smiled upon realizing that he had indeed been taught what he most needed to know: patience, self-discipline, and internal power. (Figure 1-2)

1. Chi Flow Assists the Heart

This system regards the heart as both a muscle and a vital organ. Taoists would agree that even a strong heart should never be overworked. The heart never truly rests from the time it begins to beat. As blood carries oxygen and nutrients throughout the body, its circulation can be a burden to the heart if physical stress remains constant. (Figure 1-3) When energized with Chi, however, the blood becomes lighter and easier to move, allowing the heart to work less and maintain a higher energy level. The practice of Bone Marrow Nei Kung helps to develop the Chi flow while improving the heart's capabilities.

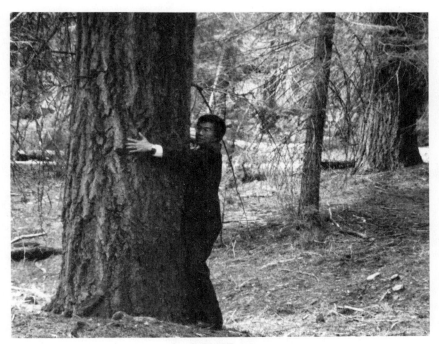

FIGURE 1-2
Embracing the Tree

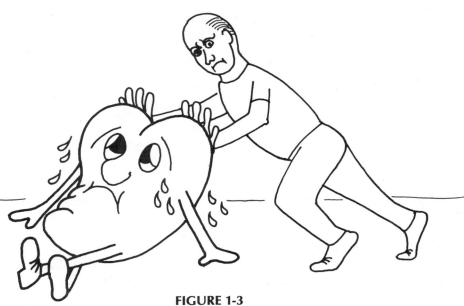

FIGURE 1-3
The more we push the heart, the more we exhaust its energy

2. The Mind Moves Energy

The flow of Chi can be controlled by the mind to greatly reduce the work of the heart. If, for example, your hands and legs are cold, you may concentrate and direct the Chi to flow with the blood to warm those areas. "Pulsing" is a meditation technique used to make the blood flow with less dependence on the pumping of the heart. Pulsing can direct the Chi to help circulate blood throughout the body. The method amplifies the pulse at the crown and at the perineum so that blood can be directed from all three points rather than from the heart alone. This practice is used to assist the heart in Bone Marrow Nei Kung, and it exemplifies some of the physical manifestations of meditation.

3. Developing Chi Pressure

Chi pressure is important in Bone Marrow Nei Kung as energy is compressed into the cavities of the body to provide for the vital functions of the internal system. A healthy body has a Chi pressure level of about fourteen and seven-tenths pounds per square inch. When we are sick, or become old, this pressure decreases, and the body reacts like a car tire losing air. (Figure 1-4) Bone Marrow Nei Kung employs special breathing techniques, first introduced in Iron Shirt I, to double the Chi pressure in and around the organs and glands. This is like creating an additional, powerful heart to improve one's internal capabilities. The Chi pressure also protects the body from internal injury resulting from external forces.

4. Circulating and Storing Chi through Acupuncture Meridians

During the development of acupuncture, the Taoist masters discovered a network of pathways through which energy could be distributed to all areas of the body. Modern science describes these pathways as conductors of electric current with storage compartments of electromagnetic energy. The Taoists simply referred to them as routes, meridians, or channels. As Chi flows through each channel, it energizes the particular organs associated with that channel. In the practice of Bone Marrow Nei Kung, energy is conducted through these acupuncture meridians to enhance the organs, glands, fasciae, muscles, and bones, rejuvenating the entire body.

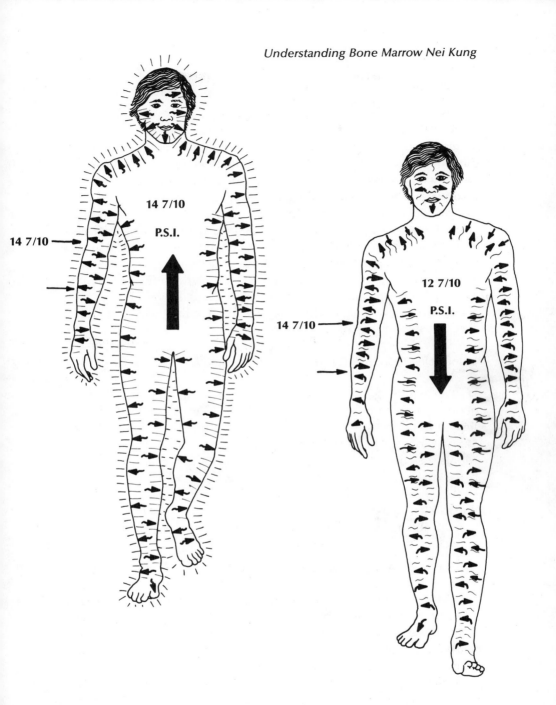

FIGURE 1-4
A healthy body has an internal pressure of fourteen and seven-tenths pounds of
pressure per square inch (P.S.I.) Any reduction of this pressure increases the
chances of illness and overall weakness

5. Chi and the Crystalline Properties of Bones in Western Research

Dr. Gabriel Cousens has compiled many documented studies pertaining to the crystalline properties of the human bone structure. In his book, *Spiritual Nutrition and the Rainbow Diet*, he reports that bones can receive and emanate electromagnetic fields in the same manner as other crystalline structures. These fields can affect cell nutrition, cell functions, enzyme activity, energy transfer, and many other internal activities. Bone-generated electromagnetic fields relate directly to the assimilation of nutrient energy, which means that they affect our intake of energy from external sources such as food.

The fact that externally created electromagnetic fields can affect the crystalline properties of bones might explain how a small electrical current can be used to help the bones heal themselves. Calcium lost in osteoporosis has been replaced through this technique. It is unknown how this process works, but Taoists suggested its use long before electrical impulses could be generated by anything other than the body.

These findings may someday help the West to accept Taoist ideas about the use of energy as a healing tool. Research has already confirmed the effects of electromagnetic energy on bone functions, and Taoist concepts seem to intrigue Western medicine as electrical current is now being used to heal bones. (Bone Breathing and Bone Compression exemplify how this process was originally employed.) It would appear that Taoist practices offer an approach to healing similar to electromedicine, but in fact these practices actually prevent bone problems and other disorders from ever occurring.

6. Taoist Practices Strengthen the Immune System

Western science is conducting studies to ascertain the effects of Taoist methods—and those of various other disciplines—on the immune system. Research is being conducted in the fields of psycho-neuroimmunology, behavioral medicine, and movement therapy. So far there is no evidence that would establish any single discipline as a comprehensive approach to strengthening the immune system. One may conclude, however, that self-induced healing, as advocated by Taoists, is creating a foundation for such a program. This ancient approach has illuminated the link between the immune system and the power of the mind. The "Inner Smile" meditation clearly exemplifies the benefits of this connection. (Figure 1-5 (a) and (b))

46

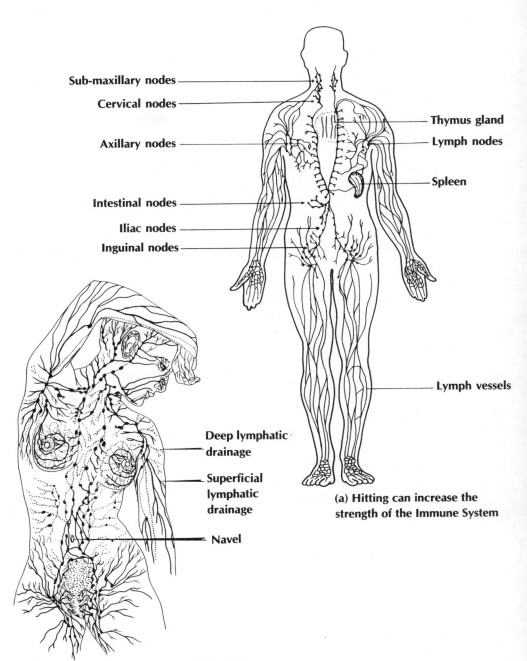

Sub-maxillary nodes

Cervical nodes

Axillary nodes

Intestinal nodes

Iliac nodes

Inguinal nodes

Thymus gland

Lymph nodes

Spleen

Lymph vessels

Deep lymphatic drainage

Superficial lymphatic drainage

Navel

(a) Hitting can increase the strength of the Immune System

(b) The superficial and deep lymphatic drainage of the head, arms, and torso is increased by Hitting with Rattan Sticks

FIGURE 1-5
The Immune System

7. Cultivation of Sexual Energy Leads to Personal Power

Nurturing Ching Chi through Bone Marrow Nei Kung and Healing Love practices eventually brings great personal power as sexual energy begins to radiate from the body. This energy has a magnetic quality that attracts people. It nourishes those who do not have the knowledge to store Chi for themselves, but it can also attract those who have other energies to share. In other words, you may attract the yin counterpart to your yang energy, or vice versa. When such a meeting occurs, the abundance of sexual energy becomes even more important as it can be shared to create the foundation for a spiritual bonding. Two can share in this joy when the energies overflow from both participants.

8. Developing the Spirit Body with Internal Energy

During its journey through the Microcosmic Orbit, sexual energy transforms into life force energy, which ultimately transforms into spiritual energy. This final transformation yields the raw material for the creation of a "spirit body," which is used as a vehicle for the ethereal being within each of us. (Figure 1-6) This metaphysical part of ourselves is vulnerable unless we use our energies to fortify it. By creating the spirit body, the spirit is strengthened and given a safe means of transportation to and from other realms. The cultivation of this vehicle leads to the ultimate experience of the Tao.

E. CHAPTER SUMMARY

1. Bone Marrow Nei Kung was created to fulfill several functions leading to the rejuvenation of the bone marrow and the enhancement of the blood:
   a. Breathing in energy from external sources
   b. Drawing in and circulating sexual energy throughout the body
   c. Vibrating the bones to open their pores for energy absorption
   d. Compressing the combined energies into the bones to eliminate fat
   e. Enhancing the nervous and lymphatic systems while detoxifying the skin

2. These functions are served by the following practices:
   a. Bone Breathing draws in external energy through the fingertips and the toes and circulates it throughout the body.

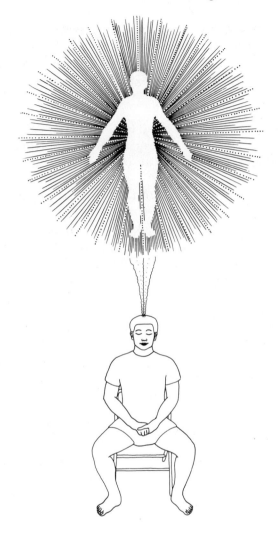

FIGURE 1-6
The Spirit Body

b. Bone Compression combines external and sexual energies while compressing them into the bones.

c. The Sexual Energy Massage releases Ching Chi upward into the body so that it can be used to regrow the bone marrow.

d. The first Hitting form creates vibrations which open the pores of the bones to absorb external and sexual energies as the body detoxifies.

49

e. The second Hitting form improves the nervous system and the external aspects of the body as the skin detoxifies.

f. Chi Weight Lifting releases the highest concentration of sexual energy and hormones as it strengthens the fasciae surrounding the organs.

3. Four practices must be used with Bone Marrow Nei Kung:

a. The Inner Smile and Microcosmic Orbit meditations energize the body and open channels for the circulation of energy to the organs and glands.

b. The Healing Love practice retains sexual energy for healing the internal organs and glands as the brain is stimulated.

c. The Iron Shirt I practice packs Chi into the layers of fasciae surrounding the organs and glands, thereby storing energy for their use.

d. The Six Healing Sounds decelerate the body after practice and release excessive heat from the internal system.

4. The energy known as "Chi" is important because:

a. Chi can regrow the bone marrow and energize the blood.

b. The mind can move Chi to assist the heart and heal the body.

c. Chi pressure creates strength and resilience within the body.

d. Chi can strengthen the immune system, increase one's sexual and personal power, and enhance one's spiritual perspectives.

Chapter Two

HEALTHY BONES: BONE BREATHING AND BONE COMPRESSION

There are many health benefits to Bone Breathing and Bone Compression. These techniques can be used independently of the other Bone Marrow Nei Kung exercises. They can be practiced anywhere, even while riding on a bus or waiting on line, as long as there are no serious distractions. They help to remove fat from the bone marrow and create space for the marrow to grow, thereby increasing one's ability to produce blood cells. They also relieve tension in the muscles, permitting Chi and blood to circulate freely.

The spinal cord benefits from the energy Bone Breathing draws into it. People with back problems can concentrate on Bone Breathing in and around the spinal cord to relieve discomfort in the area while strengthening the back. Back tension and pain are released from the body as the vertebrae are gently separated and cushioned by the Chi. The overall results will be a healthier body with increased internal power.

Cosmic energy constantly comes to the earth in the form of extremely fine particles produced as stars evolve through their life cycles. All forms of life on earth, including humans, depend on this energy which is absorbed through breathing and assimilating food.

The use of external energy to fortify the bones is a meditative process which uses long, deep breathing cycles. Bone Breathing draws Chi in through the fingertips, the toes, and all of the protruding bones, spreading it throughout the skeletal structure. (Figure 2-1) This energy is then compressed into the bones through muscular contractions, forcing Chi into the cavities of the body. Bone Compression thus completes the Bone Breathing process by retaining the accumulated energy.

51

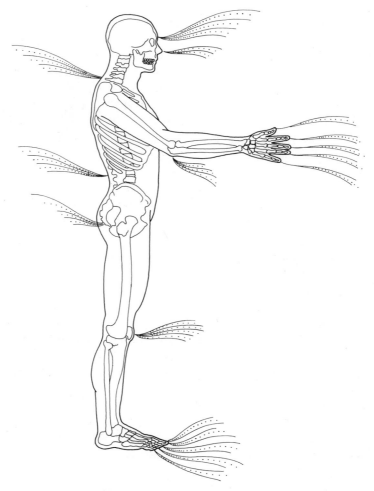

FIGURE 2-1
The energy is most effectively absorbed by the protruding bones of the body

A. THE BENEFITS OF BONE BREATHING AND BONE COMPRESSION

1. Healthy Bones and the Production of Blood

Red blood cells are produced by the long bones of the body such as those found in the shins, thighs and arms. They circulate oxygen and eliminate carbon dioxide. White blood cells are produced by the flat bones such as the pelvis, sternum, scapulae and skull. They are vital to the body's defense system. Both red and white blood cells are produced in the marrow of the bones; which type of cells are produced depends on the type of marrow that predominates.

Healthy bones contain more red marrow, which produces blood cells. Yellow bone marrow also exists, producing fat which accumulates as the body ages. When neglected through lack of exercise, this accumulation can decrease the proportion of red marrow crucial to the production of blood. Although yellow marrow can also produce blood cells, healthy blood production is contingent upon a higher proportion of red marrow in the bones and less fat. For this reason, Bone Marrow Nei Kung practitioners always seek to increase the growth of red marrow while eliminating fat. (Figure 2-2)

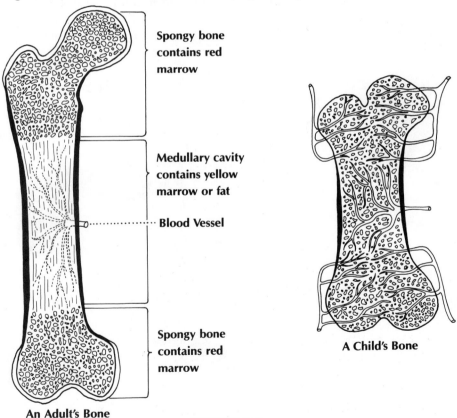

Spongy bone contains red marrow

Medullary cavity contains yellow marrow or fat

Blood Vessel

Spongy bone contains red marrow

An Adult's Bone

A Child's Bone

FIGURE 2-2
The bones of a child are made up exclusively of red marrow with abundant blood vessels, while adult bones have red marrow at the extremeties and a central area containing fat (yellow marrow)

2. Improving the Heart Function

In the advanced practice of Bone Breathing, the process of "Pulsing" can relieve the heart of excessive work while increasing circulation in other parts of the body. Pulsing uses the mind to amplify the pulse in the crown and perineum points. The pulse from these outer regions can then be used to move the Chi, and thereby move the blood. Through this process, the heart uses less force in its pumping action, and there is less need to tap its energy reserves.

You can also feel the pulse from the outer regions and mentally slow it down at the source. Hold either wrist between the thumb and forefinger of the opposite hand to determine the pulse. Then, by mentally decreasing the number of beats per second in the crown and perineum points, you can decrease the rate of the heart's pumping action. Both methods of reducing the heart's work can be applied simultaneously. Simply increase the strength of each beat from the crown and perineum as you slow down the heart rate.

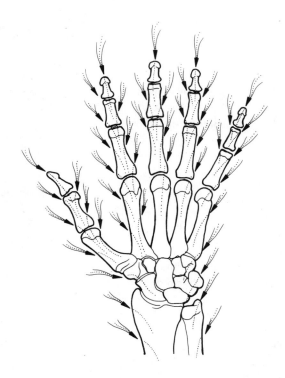

FIGURE 2-3
Bones are extremely porous and are always "breathing"

B. AN OVERVIEW OF BONE BREATHING AND BONE COMPRESSION

Bones are extremely porous, and they are always "breathing." (Figure 2-3) The pores allow the passage of oxygen, blood, and nutrition through the bones in the same way a sponge absorbs and releases water. Bone Breathing draws external Chi in through the skin, muscles, and tendons to be combined with sexual energy and compressed into the marrow of the bones through the Bone Compression practice. This process uses the combined energies to create the heat necessary to burn the fat out of the marrow. (Figure 2-4)

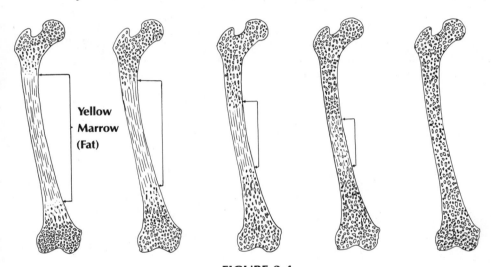

Yellow Marrow (Fat)

FIGURE 2-4
Prolonged Bone Marrow Nei Kung practice helps to clear the fat from the bones, nurturing the regrowth of the red marrow

1. Bone Breathing

Look closely at the skeletal structure illustrated in Figure 2-5. Prepare to draw in external Chi through the tips of your fingers and toes as you breathe in and out through them. (Figure 2-6) Energy can be drawn in through the hands and feet by fostering a sense of coolness in them. This imagined cold will actually attract warm external energies. When you inhale through the fingers, the feeling is usually cool. When you exhale, the feeling is warm. Once you have established the feeling of the energy in your fingers, use your mind to guide the Chi upward into the limbs and the body as you inhale.

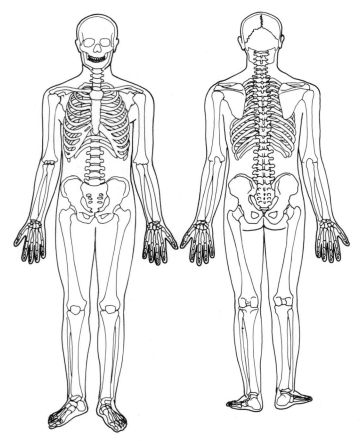

FIGURE 2-5
The Skeletal Structure

Each time you exhale and release the Chi, you can draw it back further into each limb with more force like a battering ram. This opens the channels of the arms and legs so that more energy can be drawn into the body. By the time the energy passes beyond your elbows and knees, however, you may not feel that you can expel the energy as your limbs may seem longer than your breath cycles. A physical feeling will indicate that the energy is being retained.

NOTE: These techniques should initially be practiced from a seated position until you are able to draw the energy while standing in the "Embracing the Tree" posture. (See Appendix 1.) If possible, try to keep your feet bare since shoes and socks impede the drawing of energy through the lower limbs.

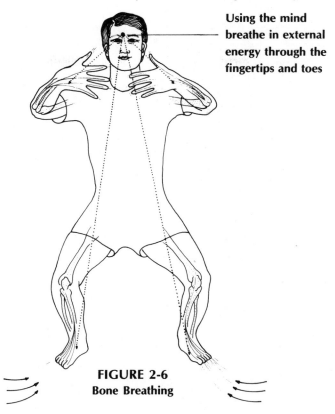

Using the mind breathe in external energy through the fingertips and toes

FIGURE 2-6
Bone Breathing

a. Respiration through the Fingers: In the first stage of Bone Breathing, use lower abdominal breathing to draw energy in through the fingertips. Then gradually move the Chi up through the hands, arms, shoulders and scapulae, up to the skull, and then back down the spinal column to the middle back. (Figure 2-7) Mentally create a cool feeling in the hands to attract the warm external Chi. Briefly hold each breath before releasing the Chi as you exhale. Draw the energy in further with each new breath as you continue to open the pathways for its travel.

b. Respiration through the Toes: When your feet feel cool, inhale through the toes, and then by degrees into the thigh bones, hips, and sacrum. Most people feel the breathing sensation very powerfully in their legs. Each time you inhale, hold your breath—but not so long that you experience discomfort. Then, exhale down and out through the legs and toes. You may feel the energy surge from the sacrum up the back and circulate throughout the nervous system as you breathe up the spine. (Figure 2-8)

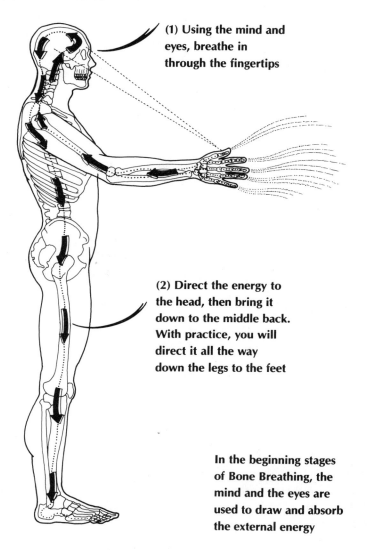

(1) Using the mind and eyes, breathe in through the fingertips

(2) Direct the energy to the head, then bring it down to the middle back. With practice, you will direct it all the way down the legs to the feet

In the beginning stages of Bone Breathing, the mind and the eyes are used to draw and absorb the external energy

FIGURE 2-7
Stage one: Respiration through the fingers

c. Simultaneous practice: Eventually, practice both of the previous stages together. With experience, there will be no need to work the arms and the legs separately. Breathe up through the toes, the legs, and up the spine in one direction as you simultaneously breathe in through the fingers, into the arms, the shoulders and scapulae, up to

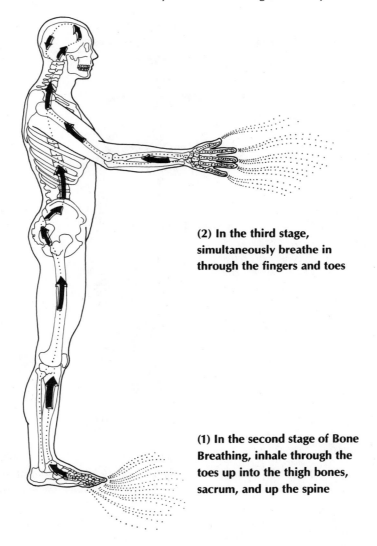

(2) In the third stage, simultaneously breathe in through the fingers and toes

(1) In the second stage of Bone Breathing, inhale through the toes up into the thigh bones, sacrum, and up the spine

FIGURE 2-8
Stages two and three: Respiration through the toes and simultaneous practice

the head, and return down the spine from the opposite direction. (Figure 2-9)

d. The energy connects the upper and lower halves of the body near the middle of the spine. The combined energies then travel back up the spine to your skull. The Chi spirals through the facial bones

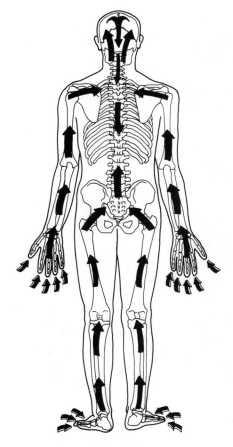

FIGURE 2-9
In the third stage of Bone Breathing, the energy is breathed in through the fingertips and toes, gradually moving up and connecting at the spine

and returns down the spine to the point at which the two sources connect.

e. After the Chi from both sources has returned to the upper spine, the energy will spread out through the rib cage and recombine at the sternum. The Chi travels from the back of the rib cage to the front. The sternum is filled with the spiraling Chi from all twelve ribs simultaneously.

2. Bone Compression

There are three steps to Bone Compression: The first is to inhale the Chi in a spiraling motion, drawing it in through the fingers and toes to surround the bones of the arms, legs, and body. The second step is to pack the Chi in between the muscles and bones. The third step squeezes the muscles, thereby compressing the Chi into the marrow through the pores of the bones. The sequence of steps is: inhale, spiral, pack, and squeeze Chi into each part of the limbs and body successively. (Figure 2-10) (The first two steps are actually a single process.)

NOTE: Unlike the early stages of Bone Breathing, Chi is not expelled upon exhalation during Bone Compression. As you spiral the energy inward, concentrate on those parts of the body that have received the inhaled Chi. It will remain at those points until you are ready to compress it into the skeletal structure.

a. In the first stage of Bone Compression, inhale Chi into each part

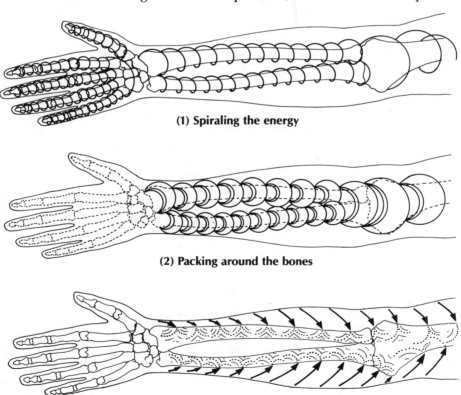

(1) Spiraling the energy

(2) Packing around the bones

(3) Squeezing the energy into the bones

FIGURE 2-10

of the skeletal system in a manner similar to Bone Breathing, but spiral the energy as you draw it in. Do not release it. As you use your mind to draw in the external Chi through your arms and legs, envision it travelling through each limb in a spiraling motion, circling clockwise through your right arm and leg, and counterclockwise through your left arm and leg. Spiraling helps to combine the external and sexual energies, while allowing the Chi to cover more internal space.

b. While spiraling helps to bring Chi into more internal areas, packing condenses it into less space. This step creates more room for the energy in every part of the limbs and body before it is compressed into the bones. Once the heart rate is audible to your "inner ear," you may amplify the pulse at the crown, the perineum, the hands, and the feet, maintaining it throughout each compression in order to decrease the work of the heart.

c. Squeeze the muscles of each hand and forearm individually after you have inhaled, spiralled, and packed Chi into them. (Figure 2-11) When you are familiar with the way it feels, work both hands at the same time. Hold your breath for a comfortable period of time as you maintain each squeeze. This helps to compress Chi into the pores of the bones. Relax your muscles as you exhale.

The resting period is extremely important. You will feel the most profound sensation of Chi at this time. Absorption during rest periods is a continuation of the compression process, using mind control instead of muscular contraction. When you release your hold, use the mind to relax the muscles and to absorb more energy into the bone marrow. The muscles and tendons should feel like cotton wrapped around your bones.

NOTE: Eventually, Bone Compression can be practiced upon all of the body simultaneously.

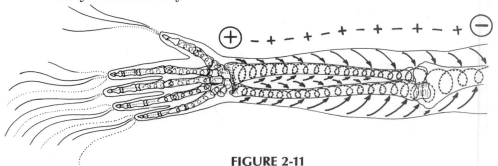

FIGURE 2-11
By inhaling through the fingertips, packing, spiraling, and squeezing energy into the bones, an electrical impulse is created

C. THE BONE BREATHING PROCESS STEP BY STEP

NOTE: The following is a detailed analysis intended for reference. Upon becoming familiar with Bone Marrow Nei Kung, students may use the summary at the end of each chapter as a practice guide.

1. Preparations

You should be certain that the Microcosmic Orbit is clear of any blockages before starting. Regulate your breathing, then circulate your energy through the Microcosmic Orbit for several cycles. (You may wish to do this from the Iron Shirt posture so that your body will feel like an integrated unit.)

Look at the illustration of the human skeleton. (Figure 2-12) Notice

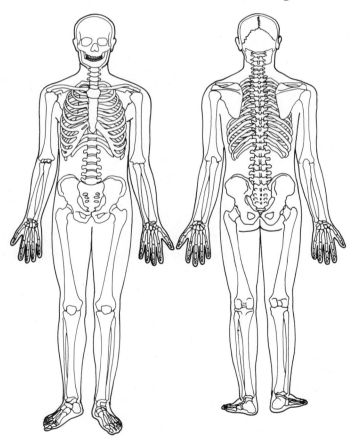

FIGURE 2-12
Observe the skeletal structure

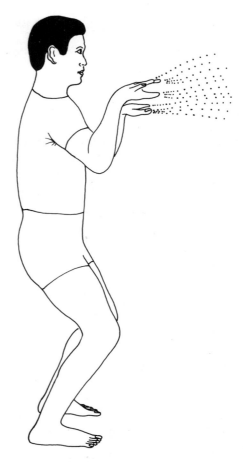

FIGURE 2-13
Sink the elbows, face the palms down, and relax the fingers. Gently pull up the sexual organ and the anus

the size, shape, and placement of the bones. Then, one arm at a time, trace your way up from the fingertips, through the bones of the hand and wrist, the radius and ulna of the forearm, the humerus of the upper arm, the collar bone (clavicle) in front, and the shoulder blade in back. Trace the legs in the same manner. This illustration should help as a guide for the energy flow in your practice.

Initiate Bone Breathing with the fingers of one hand until you feel energy moving in and out of that hand. Continue breathing up into each section of the arm. Begin your practice with the fingers of the right hand if you are right handed, or with the left hand if you are left handed. Practice using the fingers of the opposite hand, and then both hands together, moving up both arms, and so on. Similarly, practice on the right (or left) toes, and then the toes of the opposite foot, and then continue up the legs.

Some people find it useful to extend the hand they intend to breathe into, palm down, pointing outward horizontally, at chest level. (Figure 2-13) This aids in concentrating on the fingers of that hand. Between each step, rest for as long as you feel the need to do so. Place your hands on your legs, palms up, and close your eyes during each resting period.

2. Initiating Bone Breathing: Breathing through the Fingers

With your hand raised, gently pull up the sexual organs and anus with each breath. Draw the energy in as you inhale; push the energy out as you exhale. As you inhale, sink the elbow down, and draw the energy in. Then exhale, extend your hand out slightly from the rising elbow, and release the energy. As you watch with your mind's eye, see the fingers beginning to breathe. Breathe through your nose in long, deep, but gentle cycles.

a. START WITH THE INDEX FINGER

The bones in the tips of the fingers are pointed and can draw in energy. Begin the Bone Breathing process from the index finger, which offers the most sensation of the energy entering and leaving. (Figure 2-14) Bend and sink the elbow while holding the lower arm up. Relax the wrist, hands, and fingers.

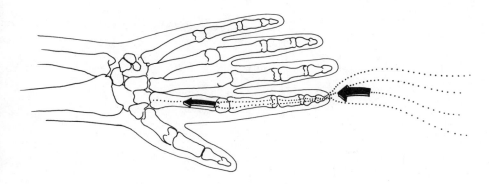

FIGURE 2-14
Begin Bone Breathing through the index finger

NOTE: If it helps you to become more aware of your index finger, press its tip with a fingernail from the other hand until you feel a sharp pain indicating the bone.

b. DRAW WARM ENERGY INTO THE COOL FINGERTIP

Sense a cold feeling in the tip of your index finger. Sink your elbow, and slowly pull in the entire hand—finger extended—with a long, gentle breath. Be aware of the energy as it enters into the tip of that finger only.

c. RELEASE THE ENERGY WITH THE BREATH

Exhale, permitting the elbow to rise slightly as you slowly extend the hand. Feel the sensation of the energy leaving the extended finger.

d. BREATHE INTO THE FINGERS INDIVIDUALLY

Next, breathe into the second, third, and fourth fingers, and finally the thumb. These need not be done individually every time you practice. This is intended only to help you to isolate the feeling of energy by concentrating on one small area at a time.

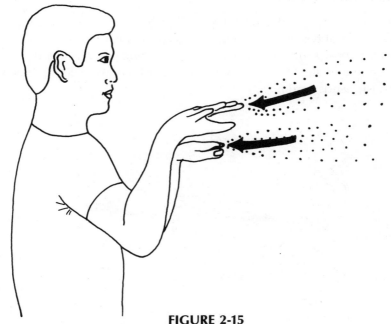

FIGURE 2-15
Draw the energy simultaneously into all the fingers of both hands

Eventually all fingers will be used to draw energy simultaneously into both hands. (Figure 2-15) The finger bones do not have much fat; hence, there is little resistance to the energy. Once you bring the energy past the finger bones into the ulna and radius bones of the arm, you will encounter more fat; therefore, breathing into them may require more practice. Now compare the fingers of the hand that have experienced Bone Breathing with the fingers of the hand that you have not yet worked on. You should notice a difference.

3. Breathing into the Entire Hand

At this point you should be able to inhale through all of your fingertips, filling the knuckles with Chi. Pull up slightly on the sexual organs as you draw energy in through your fingers. Then inhale, and hold for a while, feeling the energy as an increasing fullness, or swelling, in all fingers. Exhale, and rest. Now breathe into your entire hand, visualizing all the bones you observed in the illustration of the skeleton. (Figure 2-16) Then exhale, releasing the energy. From this point on you will always breathe into the whole hand when you begin the exercise.

NOTE: Use the Bone Breathing illustrations as reference guides. Although your objective is to learn how to feel the shape and size of each bone, the beginning stages often require more visualization.

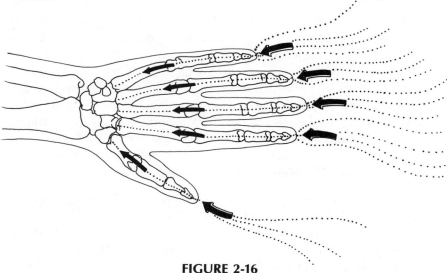

FIGURE 2-16
Breathe into the entire hand at once, and visualize all the bones

4. The Forearm and the Ulna and Radius Bones

This time send the Chi up through your hand to the wrist, and into the many small bones there. Inhale as you pull the energy up from the fingertips through the hand all the way to the ulna and radius bones of the forearm. (Figure 2-17) Hold each breath and feel the ulna and radius start to expand. Allow your eyes to close. Exhale, releasing the energy. Continue to breathe in and out of these bones several times in the same way. Exhale, and rest. Now practice breathing into the finger-tips of the opposite hand, then the hand itself, and finally into the forearm.

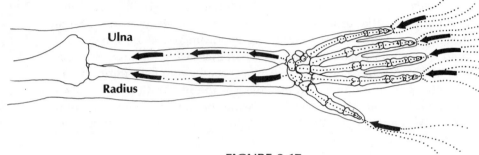

FIGURE 2-17
Breathe into the ulna and radius bones of the forearm

5. Breathing into the Upper Arm and the Humerus Bone

By now you have a good idea of the Bone Breathing process, and you should be able to expand it to the upper arm. Now you can breathe into the humerus bones of both arms simultaneously. Inhale, relax the fingers, draw energy into the bones, sink the shoulders and the humeri. Breathe through the fingers, hands and forearms into the humeri. (Figure 2-18) Exhale and continue breathing into and out of the bones. Drop the elbows and shoulders and breathe in through the arms to the humeri again. Exhale, regulate the breath, and rest.

6. The Scapulae, C-7 Point of the Neck, and the Head

Begin the exercise again. With eyes closed, breathe energy into the bones through the hands, arms, and humeri. Be certain to maintain dropped elbows and shoulders. Exhale, and then inhale again to draw energy up to both scapulae (shoulder blades) and to the C-7 point on the neck. Hold the energy there, continue breathing in and out, and then rest. Again draw the energy through the fingertips, hands, arms,

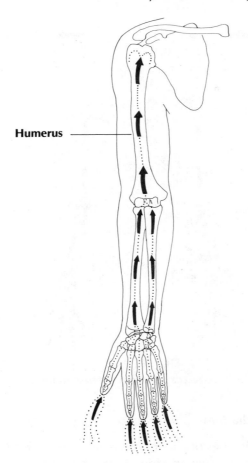

FIGURE 2-18
Breathe into humerus bone of the upper arm

humeri, scapulae, C-7, and continue to bring it all the way up into the head. Hold it there at the base of the skull. (Figure 2-19) Exhale, regulate your breathing, and rest.

NOTE: If for some reason you should stop at this point, do not leave the energy in the head. Press the tongue up to the roof of the mouth, and bring the energy down to the navel. When you are ready to combine the procedures for the arms and legs, you will not draw the Chi directly to the skull from the arms. You will first combine the energy from the two sources at the center of the spine, and then move it upwards into the skull.

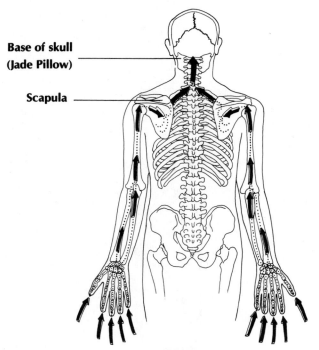

**Base of skull
(Jade Pillow)**

Scapula

FIGURE 2-19
Breathe into the scapulae and the base of the skull

7. Breathing into the Toes

Breathe into the toes one at a time. Start with the big toe of either foot, then move to the second, third, fourth and fifth toes. Finally, inhale as you draw energy into all five toes simultaneously, then exhale, allowing it to be released. (Figure 2-20) Breathe in this manner for a minute or two, then inhale strongly, drawing the energy in more forcefully—like a battering ram—to open the channels of the foot.

NOTE: Do not pull your feet up with the breath. Let them remain flat on the floor. Remember that keeping your feet bare is the best way to absorb energy into your legs. Wearing synthetic materials on your feet will impede this process.

8. Breathing into the Feet

Inhale, and draw energy through all of the toes into the entire foot. (Figure 2-21) Exhale, and release the energy. Continue breathing energy in and out. Then begin breathing through the toes of the opposite

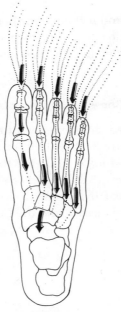

FIGURE 2-20
Inhale, and draw the energy through all the toes

foot, in the same manner described above, until you can breathe into that entire foot.

Concentrating on both feet, inhale, and bring the energy up into both feet simultaneously. Feel breath enter through all of the bones, hold it for a while, and then let the energy flow out. Inhale the energy

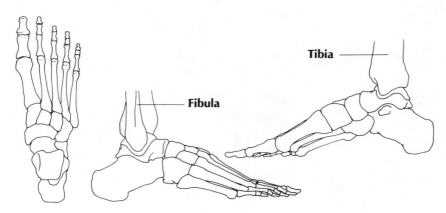

FIGURE 2-21
Bones of the feet and ankles

again, close your eyes, and feel all of the bones of both feet, up to and including the small ankle bones, as they become more alive with each breath. Return to regulated breathing, ending with an exhalation, and then rest.

9. The Tibia and Fibula Bones of the Lower Legs

With your eyes closed, draw energy into the tibia and fibula bones of both lower legs. (Figure 2-22) Hold it for a while, then release your breath and the energy. Inhale, and pull the energy up through the lower legs with more force. Exhale, and release it. Continue to breathe in and out of these bones, drawing in more energy with each breath while preparing to travel further into the upper legs.

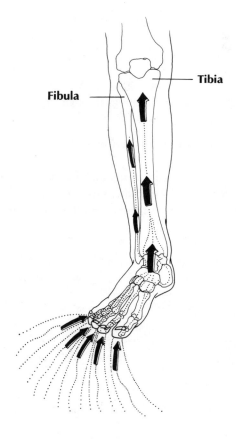

FIGURE 2-22
Inhale, and draw the energy all the way into the fibula and tibia bones

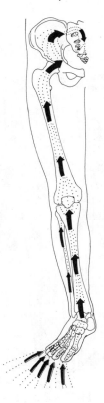

FIGURE 2-23
Inhale, and draw the energy all the way into the sacrum

10. The Thigh Bones, Hips, and Sacrum

Inhale from the tips of the toes all the way through the feet, ankles, tibia, and fibula bones of both legs, and draw energy up to each leg's femur, or thigh bone. Hold your breath and the energy there, and then exhale. If you cannot feel the connection between the thigh bones and the hips, look at the illustration to avoid any confusion. Also note how the hip bones connect to the sacrum. Breathe up the entire length of both legs into the hip bones and into the sacrum. (Figure 2-23) Exhale, and rest.

11. Breathing into the Hands and Feet Together

In the next step of Bone Breathing, breathe into both hands and feet simultaneously. Inhale all the way up to the shoulders and scapulae through the arms, and up to the thigh and hip bones

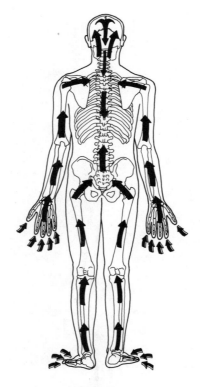

FIGURE 2-24
Breathe in through the hands and feet simultaneously, and combine the energy at the middle of the spine

through the legs. Hold your breath, then exhale. With practice you will learn to divide your concentration between the absorption points of the feet and hands. Combine the energy at the middle of the spine. (Figure 2-24)

12. Breathing into the Sacrum and Spine

You may wish to stand during this step of the exercise. This will help energy travel up the spine. The "Embracing the Tree" posture of Iron Shirt I is useful here. The next point to breathe into from the legs is the plate-like structure at the base of the spine referred to as the sacrum. Feel the sacrum with your fingertips. As you breathe in again up through the legs and hip bones, draw the energy from the legs together at the sacrum point.

When energy reaches this point it may take off on its own, travelling the length of the spine. If the energy does not travel up the spine spontaneously, continue to breathe up the back until the spine receives energy from the sacrum. Then include the breathed-in Chi from the length of the arms. The two energies of the arms and legs should meet beneath the shoulder blades on the spine at T-11. Combine the two energies, sending them to the shoulders, to C-7, and into the head. (Figure 2-25)

13. Breathing into the Collarbone, Sternum, and Ribs

Locate the collarbone at the front of the body and the sternum, or breastbone, at the middle of the chest where the ribs are attached.

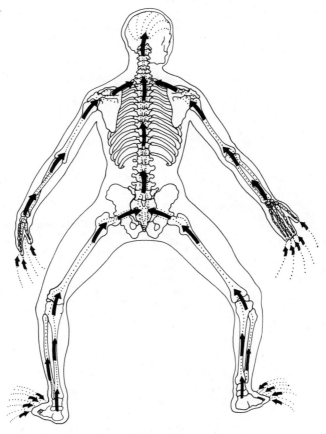

FIGURE 2-25
Breathing into the sacrum and spine

75

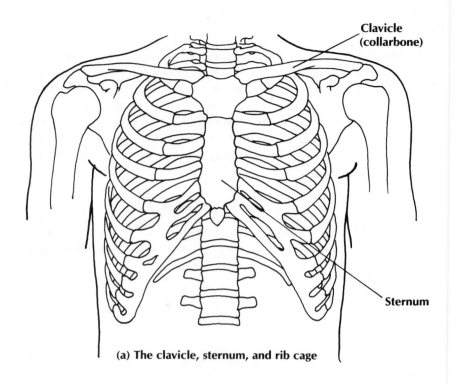

(a) The clavicle, sternum, and rib cage

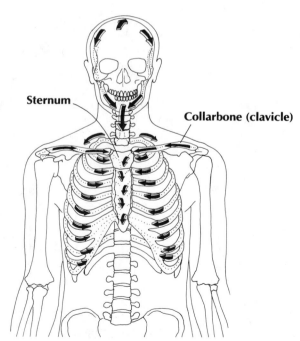

(b) Breathing into the collarbone, sternum, and ribs

FIGURE 2-26

(Figure 2-26(a)) Feel the way the ribs arch away from the sternum in the front and connect to the spine in the back. These are difficult structures to breathe Chi into requiring your utmost concentration.

The combined Chi from the legs and the arms is first breathed into the cranial area before it is sent back down the spinal cord to the point at which the ribs extend. Spiral Chi throughout the head and facial bones. From there, bring it into the spine and collarbone, spreading energy throughout the ribs, finally reaching the sternum. (Figure 2-26(b))

D. THE BONE COMPRESSION PROCESS STEP BY STEP

The sequence used in Bone Breathing is also used in Bone Compression. The circulation of the energy differs, however, in that it spirals around the bones while rising into each limb. Then, as it accumulates, the energy is packed tightly and compressed into the bones. Refer to Figure 2-27(a) for an illustration of what spiraling might look like to your inner eye. Figure 2-27(b) and (c) demonstrate the difference between packing and squeezing: One process pulls Chi between the muscles and bones; the other compresses it into the bones. As stated earlier, packing is a mental process, while squeezing is a physical process.

1. One Hand and Forearm

Practice with either hand alone first, inhaling into your fingers, wrist, and then the ulna and radius bones, holding the intake from each breath. Use your inner eye to spiral energy around these bones as Chi rises into each successive limb. Visualize a clockwise spiraling motion rising in the right arm, or a counterclockwise spiraling motion if you are using the left arm.

After spiraling, inhale again, and pack the energy, mentally condensing it as it accumulates. Pull up the sexual organs and the anus as you pack energy in between the muscles and bones. Continue this process until the hand and forearm begin to feel swollen. Then, using hard muscular contractions, squeeze Chi into the bones, feeling its heat in the marrow. Apply a little more tension to reach the deeper areas of your bone structure. Hold it, exhale, and release. It is not necessary to hold each breath to the point of discomfort.

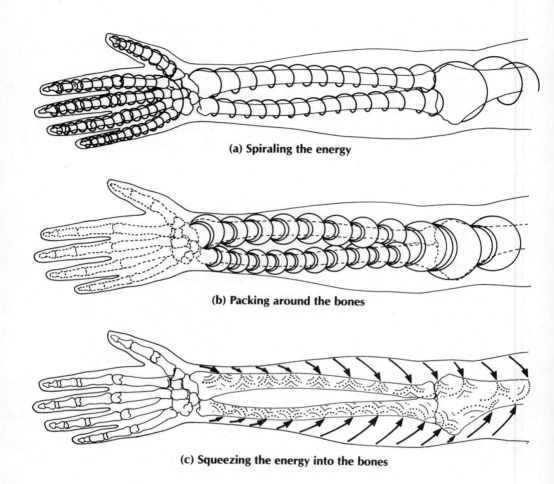

(a) Spiraling the energy

(b) Packing around the bones

(c) Squeezing the energy into the bones

FIGURE 2-27

2. Right and Left Hands Together

When you become familiar with the way this compression feels, work with both hands at the same time. After packing, hold each muscular contraction along with your breath in a long squeeze, and then release it. When you release your hold, use your mind to absorb energy into the bones. The bones, muscles and tendons should begin to feel as though they are wrapped in cotton. Always concentrate on feeling energy penetrate into the bone.

3. Both Arms Together

Now practice spiraling both hands and forearms together. Pull up the sexual organs and anus. Inhale, spiral, pack and squeeze the muscles of the lower arms repeatedly with each breath. (Figure 2-28) Exhale, and release. As you release the muscles, the Chi will not dissipate because its density is increased by packing until it can no longer escape through the skin. Next, inhale, spiral, pack and squeeze Chi into both humeri, continuing the process into the shoulders and scapulae. Exhale, and release.

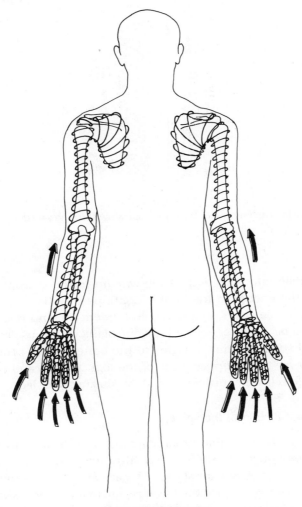

FIGURE 2-28
Spiral both hands and forearms together, and squeeze the muscles

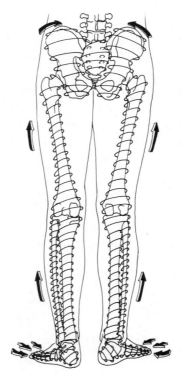

FIGURE 2-29
Bring the energy up both legs, spiraling into the sacrum

4. The Legs

Next inhale into both legs all the way up to the sacrum. (Figure 2-29) Hold the energy in the bones. Continue to inhale, spiral, and pack. Then inhale again, squeeze, hold the tension, and release. It is important to be aware of your mind controlling your muscles. Inhale energy and squeeze your muscles to the bones again, proceeding from the lower to the upper parts of the legs. Exhale, and rest. Use your mind to relax the muscles. Finish by shaking your legs.

5. The Lumbar Region of the Spine

You may wish to use the "Embracing the Tree" posture to assist in drawing energy up into the sacrum, although it can also be done while seated erect. Again, inhale, spiral, pack and squeeze the energy successively from the legs to the lower region of the spine. As you pack and squeeze Chi into the sacrum, the Sacral Pump is activated, which helps the upward flow of energy to the higher centers.

Inhale, and spiral energy from the legs, through the sacrum, and up the spine to the first lumbar. Hold the energy. Inhale again, and pack from the lower part of the leg and up so that the entire lower region feels the compression. Pack into the sacrum and the spine, then squeeze the Chi into the bones by contracting the muscles of the legs, hips, buttocks and lower back. Hold the contraction with your breath, then release it as you exhale.

6. The Spine through the Collarbone and Scapulae

Inhale, spiraling energy upward from your fingertips successively through the hands, ulnae, radii, humeri, shoulders, and into the scapulae and collarbone. Continue to pack from the scapulae into the spine down to T-11. (Figure 2-30) Squeeze the muscles surrounding the hands, arms, scapulae and spine, thereby compressing Chi into the bones of the upper region. Exhale, and rest. It is approximately at T-11 on the spine that the energy from the upper region combines with that of the lower region.

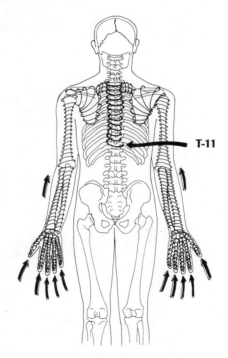

FIGURE 2-30
Bring the energy through the arms to the shoulder blades, and down the spine to T-11

7. The Cranial Bones and the Cranial Pump

From the T-11 point inhale and spiral the combined energies further up the spine, through the cervical bones in the neck, and up into the head. (Figure 2-31) When you reach the head, spiral throughout the entire cranial area, pressing your tongue to your palate. (Figure 2-32(a)) Clench your teeth and squeeze Chi into the cranial bones. This increases the activity of the Cranial Pump, which is similar to the Sacral Pump. (Figure 2- 32(b)) Both of these pumps move tremendous amounts of energy into the spine.

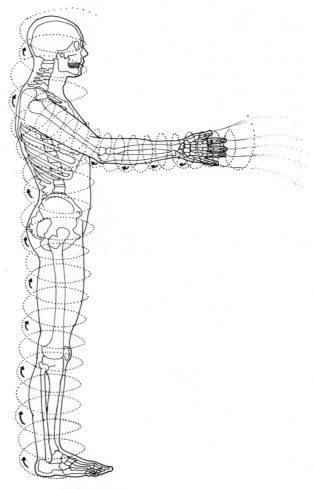

FIGURE 2-31
Spiral the energy from the legs up the spine. At the same time, spiral from the
hands to the upper spine and into the head

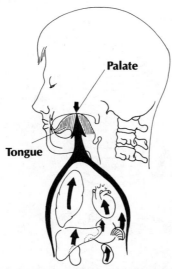

Palate

Tongue

(a) Press the tongue to the roof of the mouth with the combined power of all the internal organs

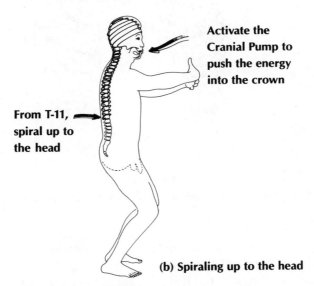

Activate the Cranial Pump to push the energy into the crown

From T-11, spiral up to the head

(b) Spiraling up to the head

FIGURE 2-32

8. The Rib Cage and Sternum

Energizing the rib cage and sternum can be problematic since the rib cage is not directly in the path of energy drawn in from either hands or feet. Success here depends on how well you have thus far managed to spiral Chi throughout the spine. When you return the combined flow of Chi from the cranium down through the spine to where the lower ribs expand outward, spiral the Chi through all

83

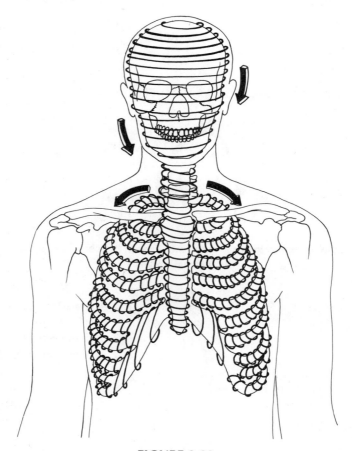

FIGURE 2-33
Spiraling from the head down to the ribs and sternum

twelve ribs simultaneously from their connection at the spine to the sternum in front. (Figure 2-33)

The spiraling will not feel as it did in the limbs; however, the same results are achieved by mentally creating a circular motion with the energy as it travels through each rib. Packing will feel the same, although there may be less muscle available to squeeze Chi into the ribs and sternum. Compress energy into the sternum by sinking your chest slightly, and squeeze into it from the surrounding muscles of the chest.

Finally, exhale. Sit or stand quietly, and feel how the energy moves within the structure of your bones. Use your mind to relax the muscles in your spine and ribs, and feel the heat as energy moves into your bones. Shake your hands, fingers, and legs, and flex your spine. Be sure that your chest is relaxed so the energy does not congest there.

E. SUMMARY OF BONE BREATHING AND BONE COMPRESSION

Although Bone Breathing and Bone Compression are most easily practiced from a seated position, advanced practitioners usually graduate to the Embracing the Tree posture as used in the practice of Iron Shirt I. This posture also suits the Hitting practices because Bone Breathing, Compression, and Hitting are later combined.

1. Bone Breathing in Practice

a. Create a sensation of coolness in the fingers of either hand. Inhale, and draw warm external energies into that hand through the fingers. Apply this to the opposite hand. Exhale, and release the energy.

b. Pull up your genitals slightly as you breathe Chi further up into the ulna and radius bones of the lower arm. Practice first on each arm, then on both together. Exhale, and release.

c. Apply the same procedure to the upper arms, drawing Chi to the humerus bones. Exhale, and release the energy. Remember to draw energy in with more force with each new inhalation, thereby accessing further points within each limb.

d. Draw Chi up through the scapulae and collarbone to reach the C-7 point and the cranium, but do not leave it there. Either combine it with the energy drawn from the legs, or store it in the navel.

e. Create a sensation of coolness in the toes of either foot. Inhale, and draw the warm external energies into that foot through the toes. Apply this to the opposite foot. Exhale, and release the energy.

f. Pull up the genitals slightly as you breathe Chi further up into the tibia and fibula bones of the lower legs. If necessary, practice on each leg individually, and then draw Chi into both legs together. Exhale, and release.

g. Draw the Chi further up with each breath into the femur bones of the upper legs, into the hips, and then to the sacrum. Exhale, but retain the energy you have breathed into these areas.

h. If you choose to combine the procedures for the arms and legs, do not draw the energy to the skull from the arms directly, but instead recombine it at the center of the spine. First breathe into both hands and feet simultaneously. Inhale Chi all the way up to the shoulders and scapulae through the arms, and up to the thigh and hip bones through the legs. Recombine this energy at the middle of the spine after it has reached the sacrum and the scapulae from their respective sources. From the center of the spine, move the energy up to the head, and then back down the spine to where the ribs begin. Exhale as needed.

i. Breathe the energy outward through the twelve ribs, encompassing the rib cage from the front to the back, and recombine the Chi at the sternum. Breathe into the sternum. Exhale.

2. Bone Compression in Practice

a. Inhale, pulling up the undertrunk, then spiral the energy up from the fingers and toes throughout the arms and legs to meet at the center of the spine. Use the same steps as in Bone Breathing, but retain the Chi by spiraling it throughout the limbs.

b. Having recombined the external energy drawn from both sources at the center of the spine, expand the Chi outward through the twelve ribs, spiraling it into the sternum.

c. The body's capacity has been reached when you can no longer spiral new Chi into the arms. Begin to pack the Chi, condensing it into the same space as the energy which has been accumulated.

d. Squeeze the muscles of the hands and arms with each breath. Hold the breath with each contraction.

e. Exhale as you release the contraction. When you release your hold, use your mind to absorb the energy into the bones through the pores of the skin. During resting periods, the sensation of drawing in energy through the skin should be felt throughout the body. Bones, muscles and tendons should begin to feel as though they are wrapped in cotton.

f. As you maintain your stance, feel the pulsing of the heart, and bring that pulse to all of the major points—particularly the crown, perineum, hands and feet. As you decrease the force of the heart's pumping, you may also reduce the heart rate. If necessary, check either wrist to feel the pulse. After you have practiced for a while, feel the sensation inside your bones. If you have a lot of fat, the feeling will be very hot. This is the fat beginning to melt. It is a good idea to practice with the tongue on the palate because, as you progress, the energy will begin to move through the Microcosmic Orbit.

Chapter Three

THE SEXUAL ENERGY MASSAGE

Taoists regard sexual energy as having creative and rejuvenative powers. They acknowledge its role in the conception of human life, but when procreation is not intended, they advocate other applications for Ching Chi. In the Healing Love practice, this energy is used to heal the internal organs and glands, increase the brain's capacity, and further open the channels of the Microcosmic Orbit. In the more advanced practice of the Sexual Energy Massage, it is also used to replenish and cultivate the blood-producing red marrow of the bones. Ching Chi is the term for sexual energy.

The Sexual Energy Massage is one of the most important practices in Bone Marrow Nei Kung. It is a beginner's equivalent to Chi Weight Lifting, which requires much more experience. The massage draws sexual energy and hormones into the body and promotes a healthy flow of blood and Chi within the sexual center. It also brings more internal energy into the genitals, and increases the production of Ching Chi. Using these techniques, men find that prostate problems can be greatly reduced, and women often alleviate the problems associated with menstruation.

The accumulation of external energy through Bone Breathing was discussed earlier as a meditative approach to harvesting Chi. For the most effective application of Bone Compression, however, sexual energy should also be harvested and subsequently compressed into the marrow along with the external Chi. This chapter explains how to disseminate sexual energy throughout the body so that it can be combined with external energy for the "cleansing of the marrow," one of the main functions of Bone Marrow Nei Kung.

A. THREE TAOIST APPROACHES TO SEXUAL ENERGY

This section is a brief explanation of the three methods used to draw sexual energy and hormones into the body. These methods provide men and women with the means of achieving great personal power through increased sexual energy. Although some of the techniques in this chapter may be similar to those found in other Healing Tao books, their application in Bone Marrow Nei Kung produces a different quality of Ching Chi. The massage techniques and exercises, such as the Power Lock, release unaroused Ching Chi into the body. This differentiates them from the Healing Love practices that require sexual stimulation.

WARNING FOR MEN AND WOMEN: Do not practice if you have any venereal infections or skin rashes in the genital area. Methods used to draw sexual energy into the body can spread existing venereal diseases to the organs.

1. Healing Love

Healing Love is a cultivation practice that does not fulfill the requirements of Bone Marrow Nei Kung by itself; however, its practice is necessary to prevent the loss of Ching Chi during all sexual activities. Healing Love also helps to open the Microcosmic Orbit to its maximum capacity while rejuvenating the internal organs and glands with sexual energy. The techniques reverse the usual outward flow of sexual energy during the orgasmic phase of sex, and draw the Ching Chi upward into the body, thereby enhancing one's internal healing capabilities. Through this practice concentrated sexual energy, extracted through the advanced disciplines, is also drawn into the Microcosmic Orbit.

NOTE: The actual release of Ching Chi into the body through the Sexual Energy Massage or Chi Weight Lifting methods presupposes that it is already abundant within the sexual center. If one suffers from chronic impotence, weakened kidneys, or any internal dysfunctions, the Healing Love methods should be mastered to accumulate Ching Chi before Bone Marrow Chi Kung is attempted.

2. The Sexual Energy Massage

For the purposes of Bone Marrow Nei Kung, the Sexual Energy Massage is the primary practice. It not only releases Ching Chi into the body, but also extracts a higher concentration of sexual hormones from the genitals to stimulate the hypothalamus, the pituitary and the pineal glands. Stimulation of the pituitary gland is believed to prevent the production of an aging hormone that ultimately brings death.

Healing Love prevents the loss of Ching Chi and rejuvenates the internal system. The Sexual Energy Massage releases higher concentrations of Ching Chi into the body for cultivating the bone marrow and stimulating the endocrine glands. When used together, the two practices constitute a safer method of disseminating sexual energy than Chi Weight Lifting.

3. Chi Weight Lifting

Chi Weight Lifting releases sexual energy and hormones to a much greater degree than the other practices. In addition, the technique exercises the fascial connections between the genitals and the internal system, thereby strengthening the organs and glands. Its practice provides the greatest abundance of Ching Chi for rejuvenating the bone marrow. It also releases maximum quantities of sexual hormones for the stimulation of the pituitary gland to prevent aging. Chi Weight Lifting is the highest level of physical practice in Bone Marrow Nei Kung.

Chi Weight Lifting should not be attempted without the proper training. After having received instruction, a student may proceed with caution to lift light weights using the genitals. At this level, the Sexual Energy Massage is used before and after Chi Weight Lifting; first to prepare the genitals, and afterwards to replenish the circulation in the sexual center, which helps to avoid blood clots. The Healing Love practices that require sexual arousal are no longer necessary because Chi Weight Lifting supplies the body with abundant Ching Chi. Healing Love must still be practiced during sex, however, unless the time is right for procreation.

4. The Three Practices in Relation to Bone Marrow Nei Kung

The Sexual Energy Massage techniques offer a greater release of Ching Chi than the Healing Love methods alone, and they can be practiced with much more safety than Chi Weight Lifting. The "Power Lock" and "Genital Compression" exercises are derived from the Healing Love practice and used as non-sexual techniques in Bone Marrow Nei Kung to channel unaroused sexual energy into the Microcosmic Orbit. The sexual application of the Power Lock is described in Appendix 1 because it is essential for maintaining Ching Chi in both men and women. Students should understand both versions before attempting Bone Marrow Nei Kung.

B. THE POWER LOCK EXERCISE FOR MEN AND WOMEN

The detailed descriptions of these exercises which follow are for learning the practice and for reference. Study them carefully. Then use the chapter summary as a quick practice guide.

1. Synopsis

The Power Lock exercise is used before and after the Sexual Energy Massage. Air is sipped in through the nose as the genitals, perineum and anus are contracted to draw Ching Chi up from the perineum into the higher centers. The three middle fingers of either hand are applied to a point located at the back of the perineum—in front of the anus—to lock the energy into the upward flow after each contraction. (Figure 3-1) Clenching the teeth and the buttocks activates the Cranial Pump and the Sacral Pump, thereby helping the energy to reach its destination at the crown point. (Figure 3-2)

WARNING: Before you begin drawing Ching Chi up to the higher centers, remember that you should never leave hot sexual energy in the head for long periods of time. Always draw it down to the navel through the Functional Channel of the Microcosmic Orbit at the end of your practice. (See Chapter Six for details regarding the Microcosmic Orbit.) There is an old Chinese saying: "Don't cook your brain." WHEN IN DOUBT ABOUT THE HOT OR COLD STATUS OF YOUR ENERGY, STORE IT IN THE NAVEL.

a. THE FIVE STATIONS

There are five points used as stations for Ching Chi in the Power Lock exercise: the sacrum, T-11, C-7, the base of the skull, and the crown. Activate the respective pumps for these stations, starting with the Sacral Pump, until the Ching Chi rises to the crown. This is done in sets using nine muscular contractions of the undertrunk simultaneously with nine sips of air to draw the energy up to each point from the perineum. The exercise then starts again at the genitals after each station has been completed, although the energy is actually held at the previous station. (Figure 3-2)

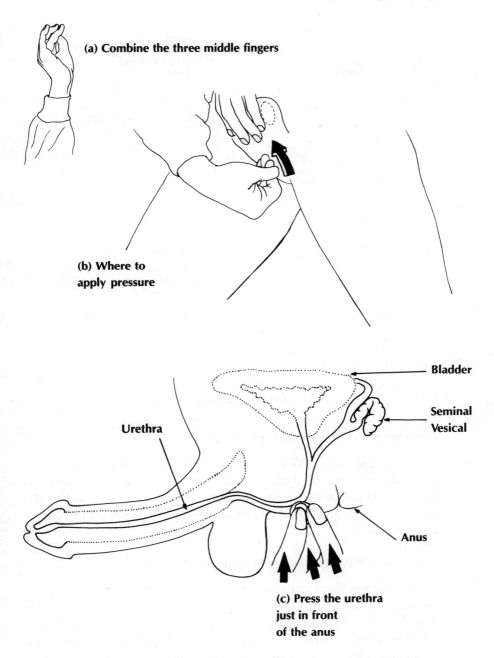

(a) Combine the three middle fingers

(b) Where to apply pressure

Bladder

Seminal Vesical

Urethra

Anus

(c) Press the urethra just in front of the anus

FIGURE 3-1
The external blocking procedure involves pressing the urethra from a point at the back of the perineum, near the anus

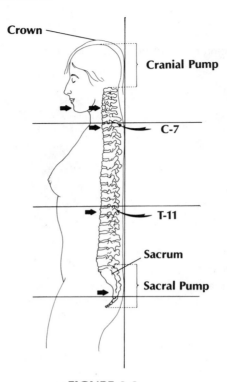

FIGURE 3-2
Sacral Pump and Cranial Pump

b. WHERE TO APPLY EXTERNAL PRESSURE

Locate the Gate of Death and Life (the perineum, or Hui-Yin) between the sex organ and the anus. (Figure 3-3) Use your fingers to find the slight depression directly in front of the anus, at the back of the perineum, and focus your attention there. Fingernails should be cut short and filed.

c. HOW TO APPLY EXTERNAL PRESSURE WITH THE FINGERS

Using either hand, combine the three middle fingers into a triangle. Immediately after each inhalation, press the three fingertips on the point in front of the anus to lock the Ching Chi into its upward journey, preventing its return to the perineum. (Women may forego using the fingers if it causes discomfort.) Release the fingertips as you sip in more air, and then re-apply them as each breath is held. Press the point only for as long as you hold each breath and muscular contraction, then release. Do not apply the fingers as you inhale because you

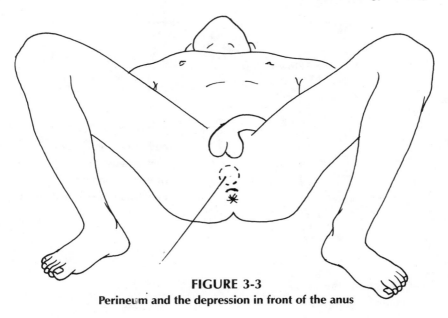

FIGURE 3-3
Perineum and the depression in front of the anus

will block the energy from rising. Remember that the fingers help to push the energy upward.

d. CONTRACTIONS ACTIVATE THE SACRAL AND CRANIAL PUMPS

Each of the five stations has a "pump" to move energy, but the Sacral and Cranial Pumps require the most concentration to become activated. The muscles of the undertrunk help to draw the energy into the sacral area. Tilt the sacrum slightly and clench the buttocks as you contract the anus and perineum to direct the energy up the spine. (Figure 3-4(a)) As the Sacral Pump is activated, it creates a vacuum in the urogenital diaphragm which draws the Ching Chi from the sexual center.

The Cranial Pump is activated by first pressing the flat part of the tongue up to the roof of the mouth as the tip of the tongue presses the lower jaw behind the teeth. (Figure 3-4(b)) Slightly clench the teeth as you pull in the chin towards the back of the head. Take in ten percent of your lung capacity with each sip of air through your nose as you pull up the genitalia, apply pressure with the three fingers, and contract the individual sections of the undertrunk. Simultaneously, push up your tongue, pull in your eyes, and look up to your crown.

NOTE: Remember never to contract the chest muscles. This can cause energy to congest around the area of the heart.

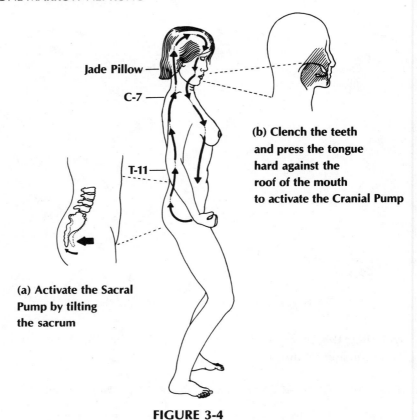

Jade Pillow

C-7

T-11

(b) Clench the teeth
and press the tongue
hard against the
roof of the mouth
to activate the Cranial Pump

(a) Activate the Sacral
Pump by tilting
the sacrum

FIGURE 3-4

e. THE SEQUENCE

Men draw sexual energy from the genitals into the perineum through Testicle Breathing. Women use Ovarian Breathing, slightly contracting the vagina to accumulate Ching Chi in the Ovarian Palace. (Refer to Chapter Six for information about these techniques.) Use a short inhalation to draw the energy through each successive point leading up to the first station. Remember to apply the fingers as you hold each sip of air. First inhale, and contract the perineum. Then inhale again as you contract the anus. With the next sip of air, pull up the back part of the anus as you draw the energy up to the sacrum. After covering these points, use several sets of nine contractions to push the energy into the sacrum. This entire sequence is repeated for each subsequent station, starting at the sexual center.

As Ching Chi expands in the sexual center, use one sip of air with each contraction to draw it up through the aforementioned points. At least one set of nine contractions should be used for each station that was previously opened. Then emphasize each new station with several sets of nine contractions. Although a week or two may be required to open each station completely, you can practice using all of the stations, concentrating more on the difficult points. Exhale after the ninth sip of air, and release the tension as you repeat the process.

f. POWER LOCK PRACTICE STEP BY STEP FOR MEN AND WOMEN

(1) STATION ONE—THE SACRUM

(a) Be aware of the sexual organ.

(b) When you feel the Ching Chi expanding, inhale and contract the perineum, drawing sexual energy into the perineum. Use your fingers to press on the point each time you contract, releasing them briefly before each subsequent contraction.

(c) Inhale, contract the anus, and draw the energy up to the anus.

(d) Inhale, contract, and draw the energy up to the back part of the anus.

(e) Inhale, and tilt the sacrum as you clench the buttocks to activate the Sacral Pump. Draw the energy up to the sacrum.

(f) Use nine contractions with nine sips of air to draw Ching Chi from the sexual center to the sacrum. (Figure 3-5)

(g) Hold the energy at the sacrum as you exhale and return your attention to the sexual organ.

(2) STATION TWO—THE T-11 POINT

(a) Repeat the previous steps, drawing the energy up through the sacrum until you reach the T-11 point.

(b) Use nine contractions with nine sips of air to draw the Ching Chi from the sexual center to T-11 on the spine. (Activate the T-11 pump by pushing the spine outward at that point.)

(c) Hold the energy there as you exhale and return your attention to the sexual organ.

(3) STATION THREE—THE C-7 POINT

(a) Repeat the previous steps, drawing the energy up through T-11 until you reach the C-7 point.

(b) Use nine contractions with nine sips of air to draw Ching Chi from the sexual center to the C-7 point. (Push the C-7 out, and pull back the chin slightly to help activate the C-7 pump.)

(c) Hold the energy there as you exhale and return your attention to the sexual organ.

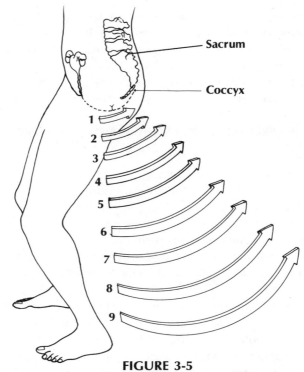

Sacrum

Coccyx

FIGURE 3-5
Collect the energy at the sexual center, then do nine contractions
to draw the energy to the sacrum

(4) STATION FOUR—THE BASE OF THE SKULL

(a) Repeat the previous steps, drawing the energy up through C-7 until you reach the base of the skull.

(b) Use nine contractions with nine sips of air to draw Ching Chi from the sexual center to the base of the skull as you activate the cranial pump. (Pull the chin back once again.)

(c) Hold the energy there as you exhale and return your attention to the sexual organ.

(5) STATION FIVE—THE CROWN

(a) Repeat the previous steps, drawing the energy up through the base of the skull until you reach the crown point. (Figure 3- 6)

(b) Use nine contractions with nine sips of air to draw Ching Chi from the sexual center to the crown. (Figure 3-7)

(c) Exhale and rest as you spiral this energy nine times outward from the crown, and then nine times inward.

(d) Finally, bring the energy down and store it in the navel.

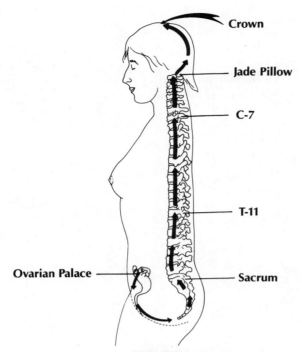

FIGURE 3-6
Power Lock guiding the energy up to the crown

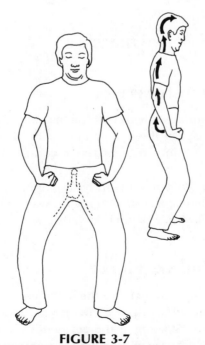

FIGURE 3-7
The Power Lock drawing the energy from the sexual center to the crown

97

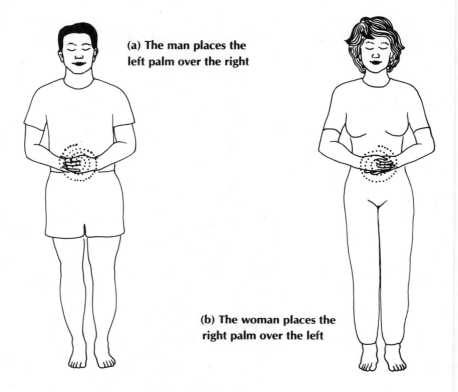

(a) The man places the left palm over the right

(b) The woman places the right palm over the left

FIGURE 3-8

g. COMPLETION OF THE POWER LOCK

MEN: Cover your navel with both palms, left hand over right. Collect and mentally spiral the energy outwardly at the navel 36 times clockwise, and then inwardly 24 times counterclockwise. (Figure 3-8(a))

WOMEN: Cover your navel with both palms, right hand over left. Collect and mentally spiral the energy outwardly from the navel 36 times counterclockwise, and then inwardly 24 times clockwise. (Figure 3-8(b))

h. MASSAGE AFTER THE POWER LOCK

The final step helps to increase the blood and Chi flow in the sexual center. Apply a silk cloth in a circular motion to the perineum, coccyx, and sacrum. Starting at the perineum use the cloth to massage the area in a clockwise motion nine to eighteen times, then coun-

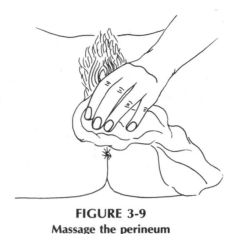

FIGURE 3-9
Massage the perineum

terclockwise nine to eighteen times. (Figure 3-9) Apply the cloth to the coccyx for the same number of repetitions, and finish at the sacrum.

C. GENITAL COMPRESSION FOR MEN AND WOMEN STEP BY STEP

The Genital Compression Exercise dynamically builds sexual power by packing electromagnetically charged energy into the testicles or the ovaries. As an expanding sensation fills the genitals, sexual energy increases, eventually reaching into higher centers of the body through the Microcosmic Orbit, as it is needed. This practice is particularly important to use after the Sexual Energy Massage or Chi Weight Lifting to replenish the energy extracted from the genitals.

(1) Loosen your pants or take them off. Sit on the edge of a chair. Men should allow the testicles to hang loose over the edge.

(2) Inhale slowly but deeply through your nostrils into the lungs, expanding the solar plexus. Simultaneously contract the anus, and pull Chi into the upper abdomen.

(3) Feel the energy of each breath culminate at a point behind the solar plexus. Use your mind and some abdominal muscles to compress the energy into a sphere at the solar plexus point. Imagine this as a ball of Chi which you will roll down the front of your body by contracting the upper abdominal muscles.

(4) Let the "Chi Ball" fortify itself with each breath, and then roll it downward from the solar plexus, through the lower abdomen, to the sexual center near the pelvis. Keep your chest relaxed to prevent any

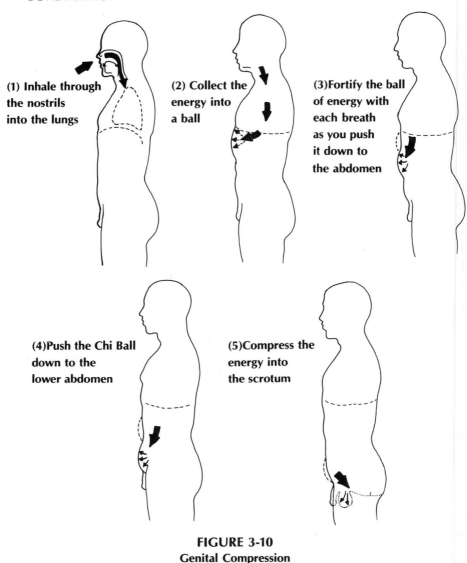

(1) Inhale through
the nostrils
into the lungs

(2) Collect the
energy into
a ball

(3) Fortify the ball
of energy with
each breath
as you push
it down to
the abdomen

(4) Push the Chi Ball
down to the
lower abdomen

(5) Compress the
energy into
the scrotum

FIGURE 3-10
Genital Compression

congestion of energy there. Use your mind to guide the Chi flow to the
sexual center and genitals. (Figure 3-10)

(5) MEN: Compress Chi into the scrotum for as long as you can.
Squeeze the anus, and gently tighten the perineum to prevent energy
loss. Eventually, only the power of the mind will be necessary to contract these areas. The muscles of the lower abdomen should also be
used as you force the scrotum to expand with energy.

100

(6) WOMEN: Compress the energy into the lower abdomen and the pelvic region while contracting the perineum, the anus, and the vagina. Locate the ovaries as they are shown in Figure 3-11. Direct the energy into both ovaries, and feel them expand with warmth.

NOTE FOR WOMEN: In the beginning it is helpful to locate the ovaries by placing both thumbs, tip facing tip, on the navel with the fingers extending downward, outlining a triangle over the lower abdomen. Where the index fingertips meet is the Ovarian Palace. Next, spread all of the fingers out from that point while maintaining the position of the index fingers. Where the tips of the pinky fingers fall on the abdomen is the approximate location of the ovaries.

(7) While still in the compression process, keep your tongue pressed against the roof of your mouth to maintain the flow of energy through the Microcosmic Orbit. Move it around to stimulate the saliva flow. Swallow deeply into the sexual center to enhance the compression. With practice, you should be able to hold the compression for as long as 30 seconds.

(8) Exhale. Take a few quick, short breaths by pulling your lower abdomen in and pushing it out (Energizer Breathing) until you are able to breathe normally. Relax completely.

(9) Repeat the exercise from three to nine times until you feel the testicles or ovaries become warm.

Remember to keep the tongue against the palate, and breathe only through the nose. When you perform Genital Compressions, especially after having practiced Bone Marrow Nei Kung for about a

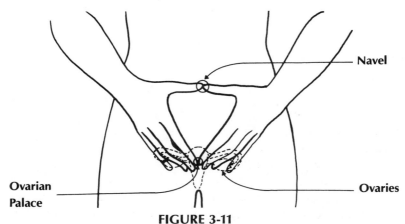

FIGURE 3-11
Locating the ovaries and the Ovarian Palace

month, you will feel more Chi being guided to the sexual organs. It is important to practice these compressions in the morning or afternoon, but not before you go to sleep.

D. PRELIMINARY CLOTH MASSAGE FOR MEN AND WOMEN

The preliminary Cloth Massage of the sexual center is an extremely important preparation for the Sexual Energy Massage techniques. It stimulates the energy and prepares the sexual organs for the role at hand. The perineum and sacrum are also massaged since they are powerful stimulators of life-force energy. First, the silk cloth is applied to activate Ching Chi. The Sexual Energy Massage then releases the Ching Chi to be assimilated into the body. While massaging with the cloth, men should feel their testicles fill with energy as they become firm. Women should feel the breasts enlarge slightly as the vagina becomes moist with secretions. Using the cloth should help you feel the Chi routes open as they are stimulated.

NOTE: After the Sexual Energy Massage or Chi Weight Lifting, the Cloth Massage of the sexual center, perineum, and sacrum should be repeated to replenish the circulation of blood and Chi in the sexual center.

1. Hold the cloth using the three middle fingers of either hand. Apply it to the sexual center in clockwise and counterclockwise motions for 36 rotations in each direction. (Figure 3-12) Men should apply

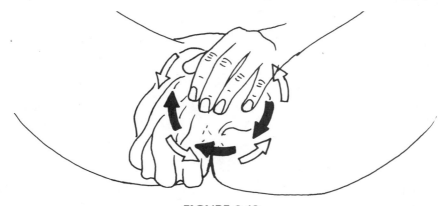

FIGURE 3-12
Massage the perineum with the cloth 36 times clockwise, and 36 times counterclockwise

102

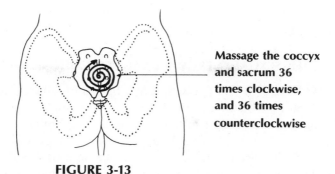

Massage the coccyx and sacrum 36 times clockwise, and 36 times counterclockwise

FIGURE 3-13

the cloth directly to the genitals. Women should cover the entire mons and labial area. Massage the vaginal muscles, pressing in on the sides of the groin.

2. Locate the perineum, and use the cloth to massage it clockwise 36 times, and then counterclockwise 36 times.

3. Apply the cloth to the coccyx and massage its tip, gradually applying more pressure to activate the Sacral Pump. Massage clockwise and then counterclockwise 36 times. Move up to the sacrum and massage it clockwise, then counterclockwise 36 times. (Figure 3-13)

E. THE SEXUAL ENERGY MASSAGE

At this point, although the practices for men and women differ greatly, the purposes and results are the same. To avoid confusion, the remainder of this chapter is divided into separate sections for men and women. The Sexual Energy Massage helps both men and women clear blockages in the Chi flow while directing energy and blood into the sexual center and enhancing the production of Ching Chi. These techniques are the main focus of this book in preparation for the higher level practices, such as Chi Weight Lifting.

The Sexual Energy Massage often causes enough stimulation to require the Healing Love techniques to avoid sexual arousal. If arousal occurs, draw the activated sexual energy into the Microcosmic Orbit. Both men and women must use the Power Lock—without arousal—before the Sexual Energy Massage to prepare for the procedures, and afterwards to draw Ching Chi up through the stations of the Microcosmic Orbit. At least two to three sets are recommended at both times.

NOTE FOR WOMEN: The second part of this section explains the techniques which are special to your needs. Study the Breast Massage described in "Procedures for Women." Section F details the "Internal Egg Exercise" as a preparation for women's Chi Weight Lifting.

1. THE SEXUAL ENERGY MASSAGE FOR MEN STEP BY STEP

WARNING: If you know that you have a blood clot in the area of the scrotum, consult a physician before applying the Sexual Energy Massage or Chi Weight Lifting techniques. Although the massage techniques in this chapter help to prevent blood clots from forming, medical advice is necessary to determine their safety with existing blood clots. Refer to Precaution 15 in Chapter Five for further information.

NOTE: In all of the following exercises, you may wrap the testicles with the cloth as you massage them.

a. FINGER MASSAGE OF THE TESTICLES

(1) Inhale Chi into the testicles as in the Genital Compression exercise. Rub your hands to warm them, and use them to warm the testicles.

(2) Hold the right testicle with the right hand. Place the pinky, fourth, third, and second fingertips on the bottom of the testicle. Place the right thumb on the top of the testicle. Hold the left testicle with the left hand in the same manner. (Figure 3-14)

(3) Use your thumbs to gently press on each testicle, with the other four fingers holding the bottom of each. Then use your thumbs to massage around the testicles 36 times clockwise, and then 36 times counterclockwise. (Figure 3-15)

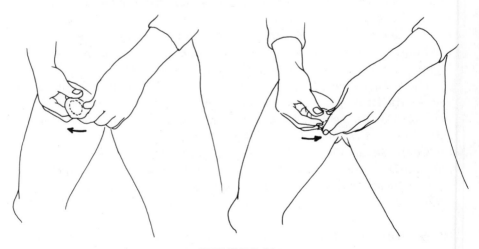

FIGURE 3-14
Finger Massage of the testicles

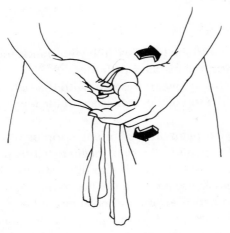

FIGURE 3-15
Rub the testicles clockwise and counterclockwise

(4) Use your thumbs to hold the testicles in place while the other four fingers of each hand roll them to the left and right, or back and forth 36 times in both directions. Draw the energy upward. (Figure 3-16)

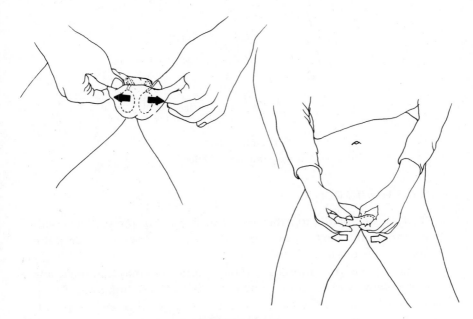

FIGURE 3-16
Roll the testicles in each direction up to 36 times

b. PALM MASSAGE OF THE TESTICLES

(1) Inhale Chi into the testicles. Rub your hands together until they are hot, and warm the testicles with them.

(2) Move the penis toward the right with the right thumb and forefinger, covering the top of the testicles with the lower edge of the right hand.

(3) Place the left palm on the bottom, cupping the testicles.

(4) Keeping the penis to the right, begin to lightly press the testicles with both hands, and then gently rub the testicles with the left palm 36 times, both clockwise and counterclockwise. (Figure 3-17)

(5) Warm the hands again, and reverse the hand positions. Then gently rub the testicles with your right palm 36 times in both directions. Draw the energy upward.

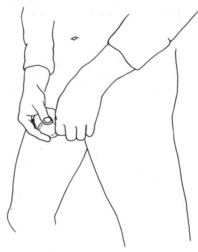

FIGURE 3-17
Massage the testicles

c. DUCTS ELONGATION RUBBING

(1) Rub your hands together to warm them, cup the testicles with them, and then trace the ducts extending upward from the rear of the testicles. (Figure 3-18)

(2) Gently use your thumbs and index fingers to massage the ducts near the point at which they connect to the testicles. Rub towards the back of each duct with your index finger, and use your thumb to rub towards the front. Gradually move along the ducts up toward the body. (Figure 3-19) Be careful.

106

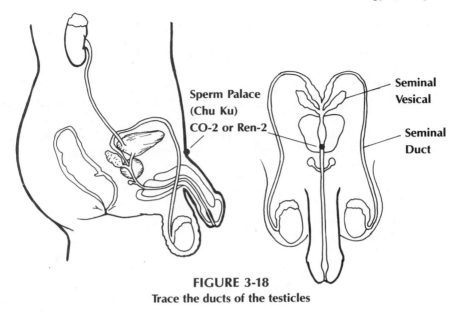

Sperm Palace
(Chu Ku)
CO-2 or Ren-2

Seminal
Vesical

Seminal
Duct

FIGURE 3-18
Trace the ducts of the testicles

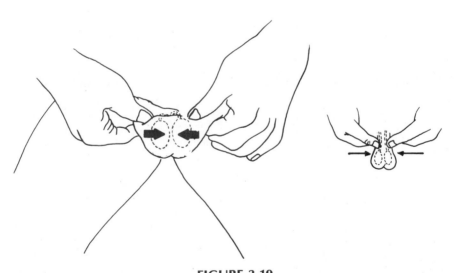

FIGURE 3-19
Ducts Elongation Rubbing

(3) Reverse finger positions and return downward toward the testicles, now using the thumb to rub the back, and the index fingers to rub the front. Continue rubbing 36 times. (Each up and down movement counts as one time.) Draw the energy into the Microcosmic Orbit.

107

d. STRETCHING THE DUCTS GENTLY WITH MASSAGE

(1) Use the thumbs and index fingers to hold the ducts, thumbs in front.

(2) Use the right thumb to rub toward the left, and use the right index finger to rub and gently pull the right testicle out, stretching the duct.

(3) Next use the left thumb to rub towards the right, and the left index finger to rub and gently pull the left testicle out, stretching the duct. (Figure 3-20)

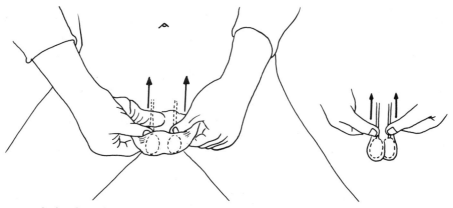

Rub the ducts between thumbs and index fingers, gently squeezing them upward

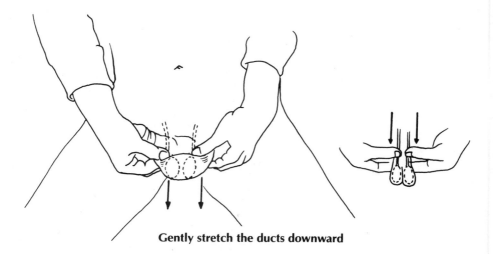

Gently stretch the ducts downward

FIGURE 3-20
Stretching the ducts gently with massage

(4) Gently palm massage both testicles, and repeat the stretching.

(5) Now you may simultaneously rub the testicles using the thumbs and index fingers of both hands up to 36 times. Draw the energy upward.

e. STRETCHING THE SCROTUM AND PENIS TENDONS

(1) PRE-STRETCHING EXERCISE

(a) Warm both hands by rubbing them together.

(b) Encircle the base of the penis with the thumb and forefinger as all of the fingers encircle the scrotum, surrounding the testicles.

(c) Gradually pull the entire groin down towards the tip of the penis as you pull the internal organs up, opposing the outward force with your hand. (Figure 3-21) First, pull straight down with the hand, and then pull down to the left and right in equal counts. (Figure 3-22) Simultaneously pull up the internal organs from the perineum, hold for a while, and then release.

(d) Pull downward in a circular motion nine to 36 times clockwise, and then counterclockwise. Draw the energy upward.

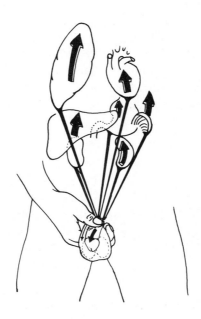

FIGURE 3-21
Gently pull down on the penis and testicles as you pull up
from the internal organs

109

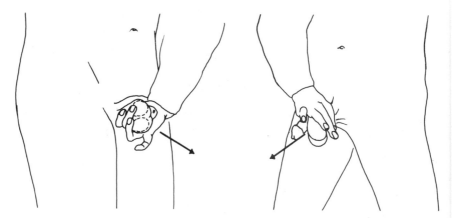

FIGURE 3-22
Stretching the scrotum and penis tendons

(2) MASSAGE THE PENIS

(a) Rub the hands together until they are hot. Use the thumbs and index fingers of both hands to hold the base of the penis from the sides.

(b) Massage the penis along three lines. Begin with the left line, using the left thumb and index finger to massage from the base of the penis to the tip and back. (Figure 3-23) Then use the right thumb and index finger to massage the right line in the same manner.

(c) Next place both thumbs and index fingers on the middle line at the base, and massage down to the glans and back. Massage all three lines, counting up and down as one time, up to 36 times.

f. TAPPING THE TESTICLES

(1) Stand in a Horse Stance with the pants off.

(2) Inhale Chi directly into the testicles, slightly pulling them up, and hold your breath. Clench the teeth, contract the perineum and anus, but only contract the testicles very slightly.

(3) Use the fingertips to lightly tap the right testicle. Tap in sets of six, seven, or nine. Exhale, rest, and draw the energy up the spine. Use the same procedures with the left testicle. (Figure 3-24)

g. RESTING

Resting after massaging is very important. Use your mind to channel your breathing into long, smooth, soft breaths. Then draw the energy of these breaths to the point on which you are working.

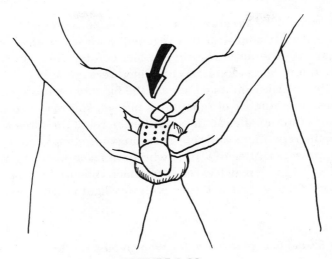

FIGURE 3-23
Massage the penis along three lines from the base to the head

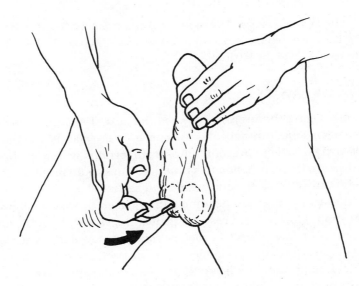

FIGURE 3-24
Tap the testicles lightly

h. SUGGESTED TIMETABLE

Practice the Sexual Energy Massage lightly for the first ten days. If you do not have time for all the techniques, try at least one of them daily. You can divide the exercises so that different sets are practiced

111

on alternate days. Practice in sets of up to 36 repetitions, as long as you are comfortable with this regimen. Forego practice, or at least decrease it, whenever you do not feel comfortable. Once you are skilled, these exercises can be completed very quickly.

After ten days you may increase the force of each exercise as you decrease the number of repetitions per set. You may also use fewer sets per exercise. After 50 days, further increase the force as you decrease the repetitions and sets, spending more time on the palm and finger massages. After this, men who have taken instruction in Bone Marrow Nei Kung may feel ready to attach the weight hanging bar to the cloth, first by itself, and then with very light weights. (See Chapter Five.)

2. The Sexual Energy Massage for Women Step by Step

NOTE: Remember to apply the preliminary Cloth Massage of the sexual center, perineum, and sacrum as prescribed earlier in this chapter.

The Sexual Energy Massage for Women is followed by the Internal Egg Exercise, which is useful in all sexual activities and is a prerequisite for Chi Weight Lifting.

a. BREAST MASSAGE

Massaging the breasts activates the sexual energy of the ovaries, which subsequently activates the energy of the glands and the organs. It is also possible to prevent lumps from forming within the breasts, or to dissolve them, by using this practice. You should find that this practice greatly enhances your health and sexuality.

(1) Begin in a seated position, either naked or wearing loose pants. You should feel a firm pressure against the vagina. To achieve this, sit up against a hard object, or place a rolled up towel between your legs. If you are naked, use a sanitary cover for protection.

(2) Pull up the middle and back parts of the anus, drawing the Chi up through the spinal cord. (Figure 3-25(a) and (b)) Then pull up the left and right sides of the anus, and bring Chi directly up to the left and right nipples.

(3) Warm the hands by rubbing them together as you inhale, and press the tongue against the roof of the mouth. Place the second joint of the middle finger of each hand directly on the nipple of its respective breast. Cup the outside of the breasts with your palms.

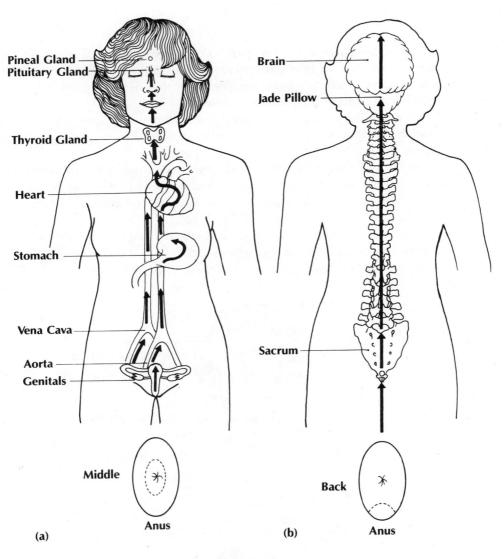

Pineal Gland
Pituitary Gland

Thyroid Gland

Heart

Stomach

Vena Cava

Aorta
Genitals

Middle

Anus

(a)

Brain

Jade Pillow

Sacrum

Back

Anus

(b)

FIGURE 3-25
Pull up the middle and back parts of the anus

b. MASSAGING THE GLANDS WITH ACCUMULATED CHI

NOTE: As you do the following exercise, combine the Chi stimulated in the breasts with the additional energy of each successive gland or organ, drawing it back up to the breasts as the energy of each is activated. Return to the breasts after each of the following steps. Think of the breasts as melting pots for the combined ingredients of Chi from the organs and glands.

113

(1) Use the three middle fingers on each breast to circle outward from the nipples, and then inward again. Move your right hand clockwise, and your left hand counterclockwise, then reverse. Direct the Chi accumulated in the breasts to the glands. (Figure 3-26)

(2) When the clitoris is energized, the sexual energy surges to the head and activates the pineal gland at the crown. Return your attention to the breasts.

(3) Continue massaging as you move your attention to the pituitary gland, behind the "third eye." You may feel pressure in the head as the energy descends to the pituitary gland. Return your attention to the breasts.

(4) Draw the activated energy down to the thyroid and parathyroid glands. Feel the expansion of these two glands as they become activated. Return both your attention and the Chi to the breasts.

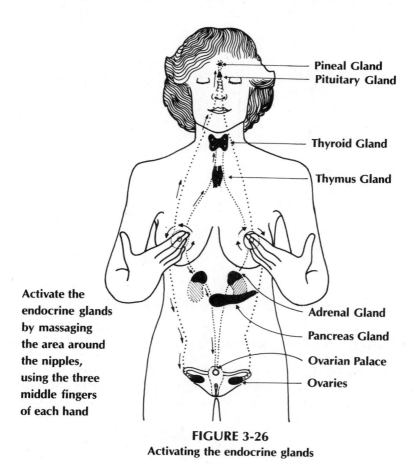

Pineal Gland
Pituitary Gland

Thyroid Gland

Thymus Gland

Activate the endocrine glands by massaging the area around the nipples, using the three middle fingers of each hand

Adrenal Gland

Pancreas Gland

Ovarian Palace

Ovaries

FIGURE 3-26
Activating the endocrine glands

(5) Continue to gently massage the breasts, and settle your attention on the thymus gland in order to activate its energy. Return your attention to the breasts with the combined Chi.

(6) Let the Chi flow down to the pancreas to activate it. Return the combined Chi to the breasts.

(7) Activate the adrenal glands with the energy, and bring it up to the breasts to blend with all the energies of the other glands. This accumulation will help to activate the organs' Chi.

c. MASSAGING THE ORGANS WITH ACCUMULATED CHI

(1) Again, rub your palms together until they are hot, and cover your breasts with your hands. Feel the Chi from the thymus and the breasts activate the energy of the lungs. (Figure 3-27) Direct this Chi back to the breasts.

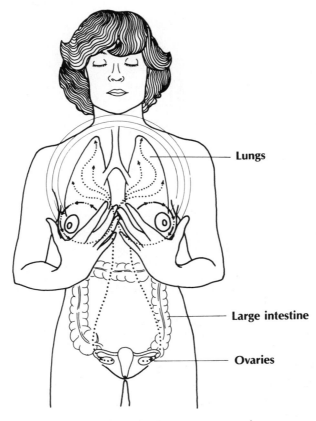

FIGURE 3-27
Chi of the lungs and large intestines

(2) Activate the heart's energy with the accumulated Chi, and direct this energy to the breasts.

(3) Direct your attention to your spleen, and allow the accumulated Chi to activate the spleen's energy. (Figure 3-28) Feel the Chi of the spleen, and direct it to the breasts.

(4) Now direct the Chi to the kidneys. (Figure 3-29) Activate the energy of the kidneys, and direct it to the breasts.

(5) Direct the Chi to the liver, and activate the liver's energy. (Figure 3-30) Draw the liver's energy into the breasts.

(6) Place your palms on your knees as you focus your attention upon your breasts. Experience the energy that has accumulated in them. Let the energy expand into the nipples as you feel a tingling warmth. Wait a few moments as the breast energy accumulates in the nipples, and then let the energy flow directly down into the ovaries. Pause, and feel the accumulated energy in the ovaries.

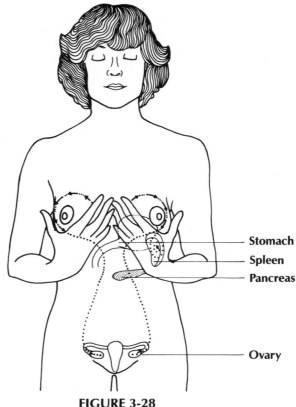

Stomach
Spleen
Pancreas

Ovary

FIGURE 3-28
Spleen, Stomach and Pancreas Chi

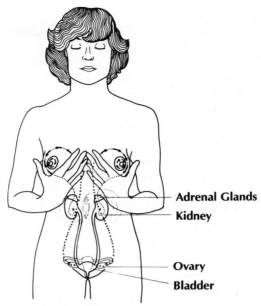

FIGURE 3-29
Kidneys, Adrenal Glands and Bladder Chi

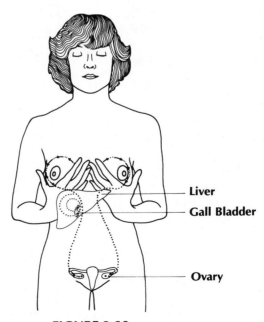

FIGURE 3-30
Liver and Gall Bladder Chi

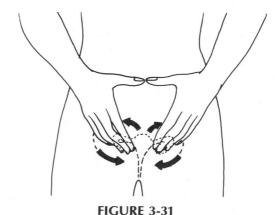

FIGURE 3-31
Massage the ovaries circling 36 times clockwise and 36 times counterclockwise

(7) Become aware of your breath and concentrate on the ovaries, breathing directly into them. Use your mind and a slight muscular contraction to move the lips of the vagina. Feel an increase in the pulsation of the vagina, and feel it open and close like the petals of a flower. When this energy becomes strong, let the vagina close in, and then draw the energy from both ovaries to merge in the Ovarian Palace three inches directly below the navel. Slightly squeeze in, tensing the cervix, and concentrate the sexual energy at this point.

d. MASSAGING THE OVARIES

After completing the breast massage, place each hand over its respective ovary at a hand's breadth below the navel on each side of the abdomen (Figure 3-31), and massage the ovaries 36 times in both directions as you did with the breasts. Once you have sufficiently stimulated the breasts and the clitoris, the warm, moist vaginal secretions indicate that the body is ready for the egg to be inserted. The Chi that is now available for your practice is comprised of energy from the organs, the glands, and the sexual center.

F. THE INTERNAL EGG EXERCISE FOR WOMEN

1. Overview

In ancient China the egg exercise was a closely guarded secret of the queen and concubines who aimed to please the king. Taoist women used it to strengthen the sexual region, thereby increasing both the Ching Chi and life-force energy that was available to them. This practice also develops internal strength and control over one's sexuality. As the egg is inserted into the vagina, the subsequent exertion used to move it within the vaginal canal increases the strength of the lower abdomen. This internal "work out" helps you develop a mastery over the Chi Muscle (refer to Chapter Five) and its functions. It also aids in gaining control over many of the involuntary muscles in the same area.

The Sexual Energy Massage is used to prepare the vagina for the insertion of the egg by training the muscles surrounding the vaginal canal, especially the Chi Muscle. The egg's use, however, is unnecessary if you prefer to initiate the internal contractions without it. (In that case the egg is only needed for Chi Weight Lifting.) The following steps also serve as a preparation for Chi Weight Lifting.

Examine Figure 3-32. The egg is used as a guideline for contractions in three specific locations:

a. The first is the front of the vaginal canal, within the external orifice.

b. The second is the middle of the canal between the first and third sections.

c. The third is directly beneath the cervix, near the end of the canal.

In contraction exercises without an egg, one simply uses the Chi Muscle to contract the three sections of the vaginal canal. Each section is contracted individually, beginning with the external orifice, then the middle canal, and then the anterior of the cervix, which is contracted before beginning once more at the orifice. The egg exercise, used in conjunction with the massage, creates more resistance within the canal. Chi Weight Lifting is the final stage of the practice, in which maximum resistance can be attained.

2. Equipment

The recommended eggs to use are made of jade. Jade and obsidian eggs can be drilled to accommodate a string passed through their centers for the advanced weight lifting practice. The obsidian eggs may require a diamond drill bit. It is recommended that any egg should be drilled, even if weights are not used. The string may help in removing the egg. Jade eggs are preferable because they are sturdy, smooth and non-porous. You may also find that jade eggs are far less

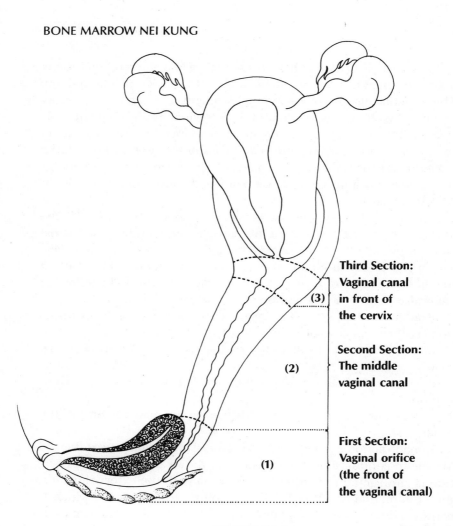

FIGURE 3-32
The three sections of the vagina

expensive. These eggs are available through the Healing Tao. Additional information on their use can be found in Chapter Five.

WARNING: Wooden eggs, or any eggs with painted or chemical finishes, should be avoided.

3. Suggestions for the Internal Egg Exercise

a. As a useful addition to this technique, it is recommended that Ovarian Breathing be practiced concurrently with the egg exercise.

(Refer to *Healing Love Through the Tao: Cultivating Female Sexual Energy.*)

b. Do not practice lying down.

c. If you have a tight vagina, or if you are a beginner, use the egg with a string to eliminate any fears of the egg becoming stuck. Ultimately, you will learn how to expel the egg without the help of the string. If an egg without a string attached gets stuck, do not panic. Relax and allow the muscles to rest until you can gradually expel the egg. When the perineum grows stronger, you may wish to advance to a double egg system.

d. Remember that this exercise should not be attempted if you have a vaginal infection or if you are menstruating. Wait at least two days until after your period is over before starting practice.

4. Preparation for Inserting the Egg

a. PERSONAL HYGIENE

Proper feminine hygiene is an absolute necessity for Bone Marrow Nei Kung. Remember that morning, preferably after bathing, is the best time to practice the Sexual Energy Massage and the Internal Egg Exercise.

b. CLEANLINESS OF THE EGG

Cleanliness of the egg is extremely important. All eggs should be boiled prior to their first use, and washed after every training session. Because some women may be unknowingly allergic to isopropyl or rubbing alcohol, avoid using them to clean the egg.

c. LUBRICATION

If the preliminary massage does not provide enough natural lubrication, lubricate the egg with a non-toxic oil or gel prior to its insertion. Be sure that the lubricant is not petroleum-based.

5. Internal Egg Exercise Step by Step

a. INSERTING THE EGG

(1) Insert the egg into the vagina, larger end first. After some practice, you should begin to increase the force of the suction used to draw it in.

(2) Once inserted, assume the "Embracing the Tree" posture described in Appendix 1, or stand with your feet parallel, at shoulder width, and the knees slightly bent. Elevate your arms in front of you to a 45 degree angle, palms facing upward, and clench your fists. Use this standing posture to practice the egg technique and to lift weights.

b. POSITIONING THE EGG (Figure 3-33)

(1) Isolate and contract the muscles that close the external vaginal orifice.

(2) Inhale slowly and deeply down into the ovaries as you gather your sexual energy. Bring it down through the uterus, to the clitoris, and then hold it there.

(3) Contract and hold the lower, middle, and upper vaginal muscles so that the egg pushes into the vaginal canal.

c. CONTRACTING THE THREE SECTIONS

As the egg is pushed into the vaginal canal, an internal sucking action is begun by contracting the three sections of the canal to move

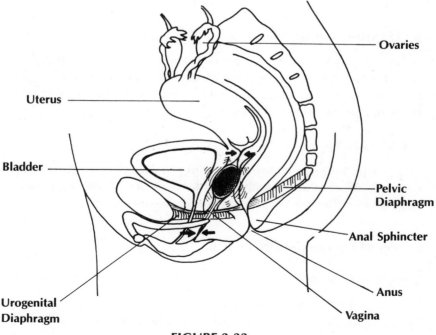

FIGURE 3-33

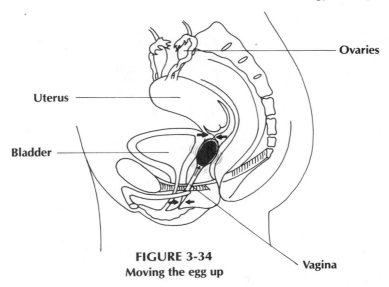

FIGURE 3-34
Moving the egg up

the egg in and out of each section. The sequence of contractions is as follows:

(1) First the orifice is contracted to draw the egg into the canal.

(2) Next, the Chi Muscle at the anterior of the cervix—third section—is contracted to force the egg back into the middle canal. At this point, the two sections are being contracted simultaneously below and above the egg.

(3) The middle canal is then gradually squeezed to establish a grip on the egg as pressure is increased to move it up and down in the canal at will. (Figure 3-34)

(4) The speed of the motion should eventually be increased and maintained until you feel the need to rest. The rest period is important as Chi will start to accumulate in the area.

(5) At this point take a deep breath and draw the accumulated energy into the Microcosmic Orbit as described earlier in this chapter. This is done after every Bone Marrow Nei Kung exercise.

d. REMOVING THE EGG

You should remove the egg by contracting the vaginal muscles to expel it. At first, a squatting position may be necessary. Try elevating one leg on a short chair to facilitate the egg's removal. If you are using an egg with a string attached, removal should be very simple, although your internal capabilities should be allowed to develop without too much external help.

123

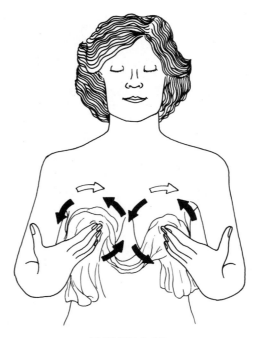

FIGURE 3-35
Massage the breasts with the cloth

e. MASSAGE

Massage the breasts and vaginal areas with a silk cloth after practicing the egg exercise. (Figure 3-35) Next, massage the perineum in a
circular motion counterclockwise for nine, eighteen, or 36 times, and
then clockwise for nine, eighteen, or 36 times. Massage the coccyx and
sacrum in the same manner using a counterclockwise motion, and
then reverse for the same number of repetitions. This will enhance the
action of the Sacral Pump and increase the upward flow of Chi, transforming raw sexual energy into life-force energy.

f. REST

Rest, then practice two or three of the Six Healing Sounds, particularly the Lung and Heart Sounds. Also practice the Microcosmic Orbit
Meditation to circulate the tremendous energy you have generated
throughout your body. Sit comfortably, concentrate on the navel, and
use the mind to move the energy. (See Appendix 1 for the Six Healing
Sounds.)

g. CLEAN THE EGG

The mucous secretions on the egg are an ideal medium for bacterial growth, so be sure to clean the egg thoroughly after each use. Jade eggs can be boiled daily, although washing may suffice. Boil the egg at least once a week for complete safety, and never let anyone else use your egg.

WARNING TO ALL PRACTITIONERS:

The Sexual Energy Massage and Chi Weight Lifting practices both require that the Hitting techniques described in Chapter Four be applied immediately after the dissemination of Ching Chi and hormones into the body. This is to help assimilate the energy before too much of it accumulates in the head.

G. CHAPTER SUMMARY

1. At this stage of Taoist practice, there are three approaches to sexual energy: Healing Love, Sexual Energy Massage, and Chi Weight Lifting.

a. Healing Love retains sexual energy, stimulates the brain, and rejuvenates the organs and glands to increase the production of Ching Chi.

b. The Sexual Energy Massage uses more of this energy as well as sexual hormones to fortify the bones, regrow marrow, and replenish the blood while strengthening the genitals and internal system. These techniques comprise one of the most important practices of Bone Marrow Nei Kung.

c. Chi Weight Lifting is the ultimate practice for releasing sexual energy into the body. It extracts the highest concentration of Ching Chi from the genitals while strengthening the fasciae, genitals, and internal system. The release of sexual hormones stimulates the pituitary gland.

2. The Power Lock: This is practiced before and after the Sexual Energy Massage to assist in the upward draw of released energy and sexual hormones. The Power Lock employs nine short sips of breath with nine contractions of the genital, anal, and perineal areas. The tongue is pushed against the palate, and the buttocks and teeth are clenched to activate the cranial and sacral pumps. In conjunction with these contractions, the three middle fingers of either hand press

a point at the back of the perineum, near the anus, to help guide the rising energy up to the five stations of the sacrum, T-11, C-7, base of the skull, and the crown. The goal is to draw sexual energy from the perineum to the crown.

3. Genital Compression: This exercise replenishes the energy drawn from the genitals during the other practices. This is not a Bone Marrow Nei Kung technique in itself, but rather a separate practice for use afterwards. The method compresses energy into the genitals to enhance their production of Ching Chi.

4. The Preliminary Cloth Massage: A silk cloth is used to massage the genital area, the perineum, the coccyx, and the sacrum. This is done before and after the Sexual Energy Massage to first prepare the genitals for the exercise, and later to replenish the flow of blood and Chi to the sexual center. This is particularly useful in preventing blood coagulation and subsequent blood clots from occurring in the genitals of male practitioners.

5. The Sexual Energy Massage For Men:
a. Finger Massage of the Testicles
b. Palm Massage of the Testicles
c. Ducts Elongation Rubbing
d. Stretching the Ducts Gently with Massage
e. Stretching the Scrotum and Penis Tendons
f. Tapping the Testicles

6. The Sexual Energy Massage for Women:
a. Breast Massage
b. Massage of the Glands with Accumulated Chi
c. Massage of the Organs with Accumulated Chi
d. Massage the Ovaries

7. The Internal Egg Exercise: This exercise uses the jade egg as a guideline for contracting the three sections of the vaginal canal to strengthen them. The first section is the front of the vaginal canal, within the external orifice. The second section is the middle of the canal between the first and third sections. The third section is directly beneath the cervix, near the end of the canal.

Chapter Four

HITTING

An interdependence exists among the Bone Marrow Nei Kung disciplines. Although some benefits are derived from these exercises individually, only their combined practice can produce the coveted "Steel Body" that transcends human frailties and disease. For example, Bone Breathing and Bone Compression work best when combined with the Hitting practice. Hitting is also used after Chi Weight Lifting to enhance the body's assimilation of Ching Chi. The practice does not depend upon the other disciplines, but it dramatically increases their effectiveness by promoting a much deeper penetration of energy into the body.

A. AN OVERVIEW OF HITTING

In the primary form of Hitting, a bundle of wire rods is used to strike specific lines along the body and limbs. (A long bean bag filled with mung and black beans may be used instead.) The wire rods create vibrations which serve to open the pores of the bones for the accumulated energies to access the bone marrow. These vibrations also shake any toxins out of the fasciae, muscles and internal organs, while breaking up deposits of uric acid and releasing tension from the body. (Figure 4-1) A second form of Hitting uses rattan sticks along the same lines to improve the exterior of the body and increase the strength of the nervous system.

The specific lines used for Hitting correspond to known acupuncture meridians that accommodate the Chi flow throughout the body. As you hit along each line, vibrations penetrate into its respective organs through the associated meridians. The Hitting device also vibrates the fascial layers, separating them while the accumulated energy inflates them like cushions to protect the internal system. The

127

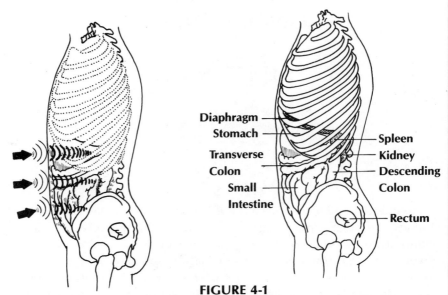

FIGURE 4-1

Vibrations from Hitting break up toxic substances deep within the body

resulting increase in Chi pressure creates a resilience within the organs, enabling them to bounce back from each strike. This rebound creates shock waves in the Chi flow from which the organs, glands, and bones can absorb more energy. (Figure 4-2)

B. THE METHODS OF HITTING

NOTE: Of the two forms of Hitting, the first focuses primarily on internal health, whereas the second is geared towards external improvements.

1. There are three methods of the first form of Hitting:

(a) "Hitting with Packing" is the most comprehensive approach to Hitting. It is the only method explained in detail here, since it encompasses the other methods. The technique works in conjunction with a Bone Breathing and Bone Compression process referred to as "Packing." This process requires that you inhale, spiral, pack and squeeze energy into the bones of a specific limb or part of the body, and then maintain the compression as you hit along the lines of that area. The process continues for each section of the arms, legs and body in succession as described below.

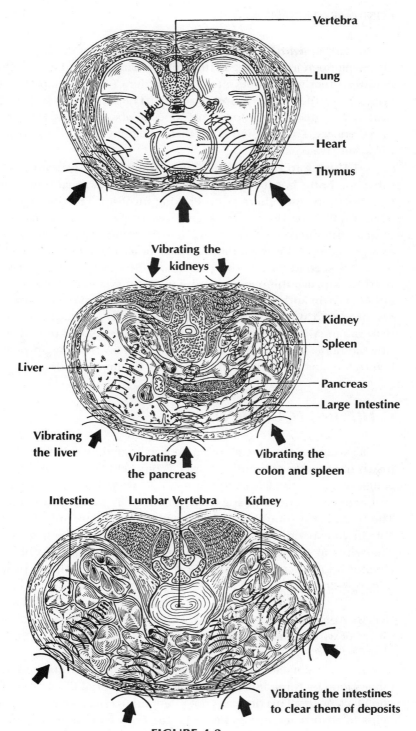

FIGURE 4-2
Cross sections of the torso showing how the vibrations reach the organs

(b) "Hitting with a Long Bean Bag" uses a sack of mung and black beans eighteen inches long instead of the wire device. The sack has a cooling effect which alleviates the problem of too much heat that arises from the other Hitting practices. The long bean bag absorbs heat and toxins while helping the bones to absorb Ching Chi and external energy. This method is useful for beginners and those who are physically weak.

(c) "Hitting to Detoxify" also uses the same Hitting lines as the other methods, but it does not include any Bone Breathing or Bone Compression since there is no Packing involved. This method relies solely on the vibrations of the wire device or the use of the bean bag to cleanse the internal system. This detoxification process can be used as a preparation for the other methods, or as a practice by itself.

2. The second form of this practice, "Hitting with Rattan Sticks," is used to improve the nervous and lymphatic systems while strengthening the skin and external features of the body. Most of the same lines are used, but no bones are hit, and Packing is unnecessary. Hitting with rattan sticks can be done immediately after any of the other Hitting methods. It is usually the final Bone Marrow Nei Kung procedure before the closing meditation and the Six Healing Sounds.

C. HITTING EQUIPMENT

Vibrations in the Hitting practice are created by a special striking instrument made of bundled wires. From 100 to 110 pieces of twelve gauge wire, cut to eighteen inch lengths, are bound together at one end with duct tape covering approximately six inches of the bundle. The bound end should be covered with enough tape to feel comfortable in your hand. The free end should be about twelve inches long. The wires at the free end should be separated slightly to help distribute the impact and create vibrations during the Hitting process. (Figure 4-3)

NOTE: Women may prefer to use a lighter wire device with 50 to 75 pieces of wire in the bundle.

The wire device can be replaced by a long bean bag, eighteen inches long by three inches wide, of strong material filled with mung and black beans. This device is not intended to create vibrations, but it helps to absorb any excess heat that the body cannot assimilate. The

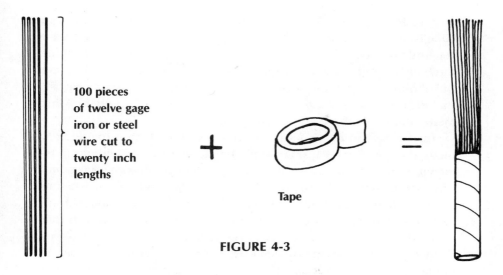

**100 pieces
of twelve gage
iron or steel
wire cut to
twenty inch
lengths**

Tape

FIGURE 4-3

bag can be used after the wire device to eliminate the problem of overheating.

The rattan sticks are cut from a very light hardwood to a length of about two feet. Two sticks are wrapped together with duct tape at approximately two inches from each end as they are held together. (Figure 4-4) The rattan sticks are used for external stimulation, which strengthens the nervous and lymphatic systems through the shock of contact with the skin.

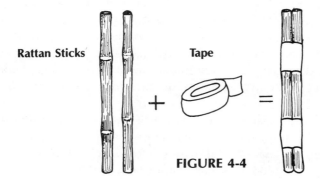

Rattan Sticks   **Tape**

FIGURE 4-4

D. CHOOSING THE RIGHT APPROACH

The format that will best serve you depends upon your goals and your physical condition, since your needs may not require a full regimen of Hitting on a daily basis. Those involved in martial arts can benefit from a complete training program, but a less comprehensive schedule is adequate for those who are interested only in detoxifying the body or improving the skin. In any case, it is recommended that the abdominal lines be hit daily as part of the detoxifying process. Include the insides of the elbows, the backs of the knees, and the Ming Men point on the back opposite the navel.

In the beginning you should only use the Hitting to Detoxify method without any Packing. Gently hit along each line without tensing your muscles, and use only three strikes to emphasize each point. The spaces between these points should also be randomly brushed in a steady rhythm. Because the vibrations of the wire device penetrate up to six inches beneath the skin, there should be little concern that some meridians and corresponding organs will miss the shock waves if any points are merely brushed over. These waves spread out as the device makes contact. Follow this with a light application of the rattan sticks.

NOTE: Hitting with Packing can also be used to detoxify, but it should not be practiced until the detoxification process works without overheating or exhausting your body.

When you advance enough to use Packing, remember to pull up the sexual organs and the urogenital and pelvic diaphragms as you compress Chi into each area. First become aware of the limb or part of the body you intend to hit. Then inhale, spiral, pack, and squeeze Chi into it, maintaining the compression as you strike the lines of that area with either Hitting device. All tension is released by exhaling after each series of hits. As you strike the body, the free hand can either be clenched in a fist or used to cover the kidney on the opposite side from that which you are Hitting. Continue this process with each successive area.

Eventually you can increase the number of times that you hit each point from three to nine as your practice evolves into a continuous, rhythmic motion. You may also increase the force with which you hit, provided that you maintain a sensible approach, since the effects of overzealous practice can be detrimental. None of the exercises in this book is intended to be difficult or strenuous in any way. After a line is hit, it is important to rest and feel the heat that is generated so that you can direct it into the upward flow of the Microcosmic Orbit.

IMPORTANT: Even if you do not intend to use Packing it is recommended that you first read Section E to learn the sequence, and then practice from the summary, which does not include the Packing process. READ THE PRECAUTIONS IN SECTION G CAREFULLY BEFORE YOU BEGIN THE PRACTICE.

E. HITTING WITH PACKING IN DETAIL

Hit gently, especially in the beginning. If you use the wire device, your goal is to create a spring-like action which will initiate gentle shock waves in the body's energy flow. (The free ends of the wires should be slightly spread to accommodate this action.) Vibrations resulting from this exercise activate the Chi and create the space for its absorption.

1. Awaken the Energy and Detoxify

The following steps constitute a warm-up exercise to prepare for Hitting. These steps are designed to stimulate the energies stored in the navel and to detoxify the places where toxins accumulate most heavily. Always hit gently, using light to medium force. Rest and practice Bone Breathing in between rounds. (Figure 4-5) After finishing the Hitting sequence, hit these four areas again to complete the practice.

a. The Tan Tien—Lower Abdomen: Hit three times the lower abdomen point located three inches directly below the navel. As you hit the navel and the Tan Tien, feel the warmth spread throughout your body. (Figure 4-6) Hit again three times, with Packing if you like, and then rest briefly.

b. Ming Men: Hit the Ming Men point—also known as the "Door of Life"—on the spine opposite the navel three times. (Figure 4-7) When Packing this area, inhale, and draw the energy up from the perineum, through the sacrum, and into the Ming Men. Also pack the two kidneys while pulling up the left and right sides of the anus. Hit the Ming Men three times again, and then rest. Be aware of the point, and use your mind to absorb the energy into the spine through the Ming Men.

c. The Back of the Knee: Hitting this point will release an enormous amount of toxins which accumulate there. (Figure 4-8) Hit three times, and then rest as you breathe energy into the bones. (Figure 4-5) Repeat the procedure.

d. Inside of the Elbow: Hitting this point initiates powerful detoxifying vibrations throughout the arms. (Figure 4-9) Hit three times. Rest as you feel the energy flow. Repeat once more.

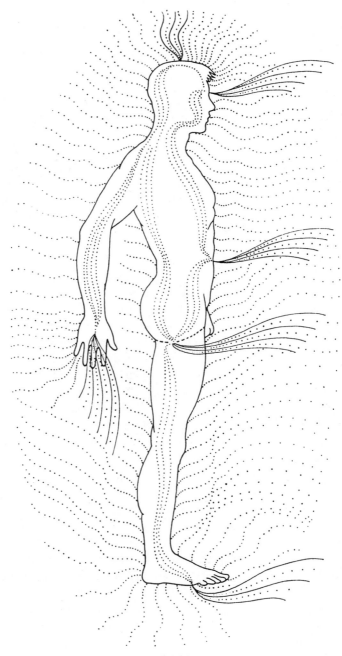

FIGURE 4-5
Rest and practice Bone Breathing, using the mind to absorb energy
into the bones and through the whole body

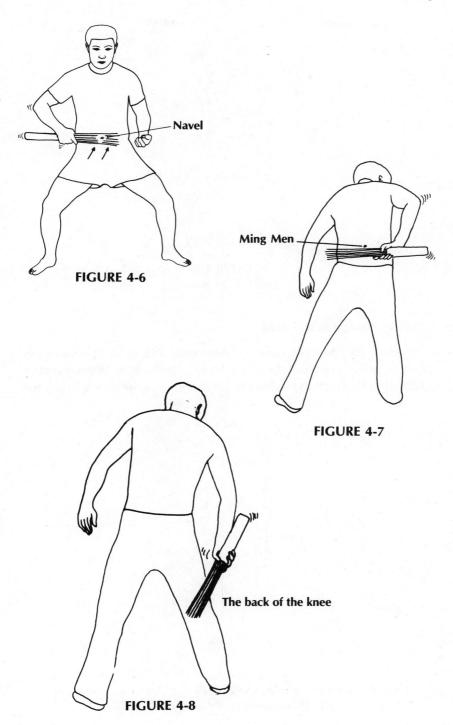

Navel

FIGURE 4-6

Ming Men

FIGURE 4-7

The back of the knee

FIGURE 4-8

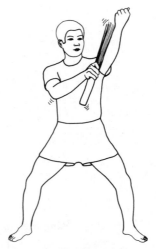

FIGURE 4-9
Inside of the elbow

2. Hitting the Abdominal Area

Practice should start with the five vertical lines of the abdomen between the rib cage and the pubic bone. (Figure 4-10) As you breathe in Chi, directing it to the navel, do not over-compress the air into your

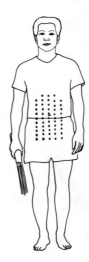

FIGURE 4-10
The five lines of the abdomen

lungs. Sip in small amounts of air—less than ten percent of your lung capacity—as you concentrate on raising the Chi pressure in the navel area. Make sure you feel the pressure at the navel and not in the chest. (Figure 4-11)

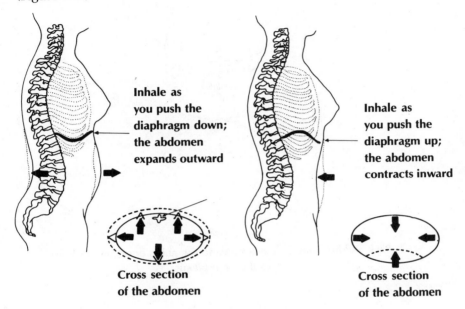

Inhale as you push the diaphragm down; the abdomen expands outward

Inhale as you push the diaphragm up; the abdomen contracts inward

Cross section
of the abdomen

Cross section
of the abdomen

FIGURE 4-11
Breathing in Chi

a. Center Line: Standing in a Horse Stance position, inhale, pulling up the genitals and the pelvic and urogenital diaphragms. After you have drawn Chi into the navel with your breath, spiral, pack, and squeeze it as you strike the compressed area three times. Apply the same procedures to the Lower Tan Tien, continuing down to the pubic bone, and then back up this line to the solar plexus. (Figure 4-12) Exhale, relax, and absorb the Chi.

b. Interior Left Abdomen: Inhale, pull up, spiral, pack, and squeeze energy into the interior left abdominal line. This channel runs parallel to the center line vertically between the ribs and the pubic bone, one and a half inches to the left of the navel. While maintaining the pressure, hit down to the pubic bone, and then back up the same line to a point just below the rib cage. (Figure 4-13) Exhale, relax, and absorb the Chi.

c. Exterior Left Abdomen: Inhale again, pull up, and pack into the exterior left abdominal line that runs parallel to lines (a) and (b) at

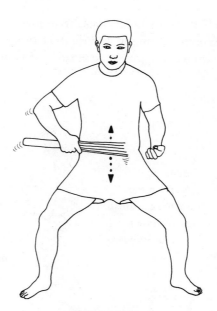

FIGURE 4-12
Pack and hit from the navel down to the pubic bone and back up
to the solar plexus

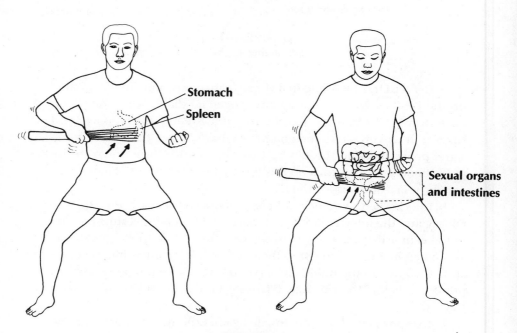

FIGURE 4-13

about three inches to the left of the navel. With the left hand raised to avoid obstructing the process, use the right hand to hit down to a point near the hip, then hit back up the same line to a point just below the rib cage. (Figure 4-14) Exhale, relax, and absorb the Chi.

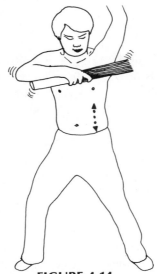

FIGURE 4-14
Hitting the exterior left abdomen

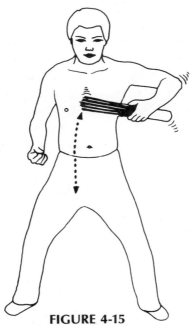

FIGURE 4-15
Hitting a vertical line parallel to the line at the navel

139

d. Hitting the interior and exterior lines on the right side of the abdomen uses the same steps as above. Use the left hand to hit as the right hand covers the right kidney, or remains in a fist. (Figure 4-15) These are lines (d) and (e) of the abdomen.

3. Hitting the Sides of the Body

The next line is located on the far left side of the body, extending downward vertically from the armpit. Raise the left arm overhead to access the left side line with the right hand. Start hitting from the floating rib—at the level of the navel—down the left side to the hip, then back up to the rib cage, continuing up to the armpit, and back down the left side again to the floating rib. Exhale, rest, and absorb the Chi. The right side line is exactly the same as the left, but this time the device is held in the left hand as the right arm is raised to facilitate Hitting. (Figure 4-16)

4. Hitting the Rib Cage

(a) The rib cage is gently hit across the chest in horizontal lines, starting from the sternum and proceeding in either direction. (Figure 4-17) Reposition the wire device at the sternum after each rib is hit, working from the bottom ribs to the top. Follow the curvature of the ribs as they guide you towards the spine.

Begin at the base of the left chest, near the sternum, with the lowest rib. (The false ribs, which are not attached to the sternum, can be hit either as part of the back, or along with the side lines which extend from beneath the armpits.) Pull up the left side of the anus as you breathe into the left side and pack Chi into it. Hit the left rib cage, moving up about one and a half inches for each rib, starting each from the sternum. Then, using the left hand, hit the right rib cage in the same manner while pulling up the right anus.

(b) The last sections to hit are the sternum and the collarbone on both sides. Hit this area from the base of the sternum, along the collarbone, and finally out to the shoulder. (Figure 4-18) Use caution while Hitting the sternum. Exhale, relax, and absorb the energy.

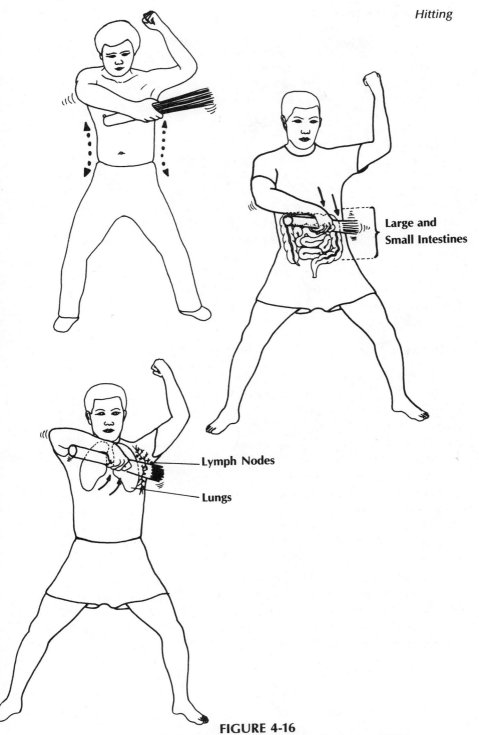

FIGURE 4-16
Hitting the sides of the body from the floating ribs to the hip

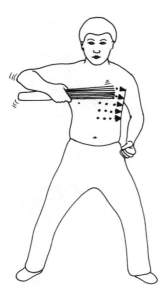

FIGURE 4-17
Hitting the ribs from the sternum outward horizontally

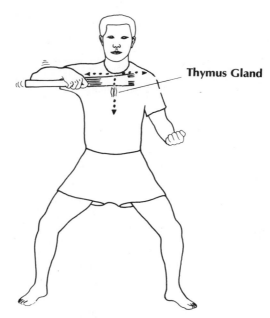

Thymus Gland

FIGURE 4-18
Hitting the sternum and the collarbone (the vibrations stimulate the thymus gland)

5. Hitting the Back

NOTE: It is always preferable to have a partner hit the lines of the back for you. This allows you to concentrate more on the absorption process and less on trying to access hard to reach areas.

a. The Lines of the Back: Hit a point three inches directly to the left of the Ming Men three times, using the right hand. (Figure 4-19) Then, round the scapulae by extending your left arm and shoulder as you sink in the chest. Pack and hit the left kidney gently, and then hit vertically all the way up to the neck. Pull your chin towards the back of the head, clench your teeth, and press your tongue to the palate as you reach the base of the skull. Return down this line to a point to the left of the sacrum, and then go back up to the starting point. Rest, and absorb the Chi. Hit the line three inches to the right of the Ming Men in the same manner.

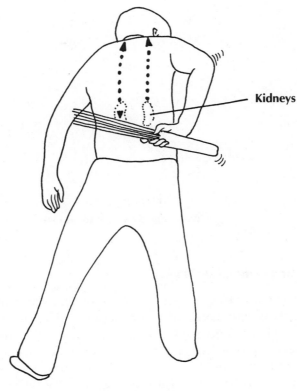

Kidneys

FIGURE 4-19
Hitting the lines extending from the kidneys to the base of the skull

6. Hitting around the Head and Jaw

Gently hit around the head, tapping at the level of the hairline, but never on top or near the crown. Then lightly tap around the outside edges of your lower jaw. (Figure 4-20) Always pull back the chin, clench your teeth, and press your tongue to the palate when Hitting the head.

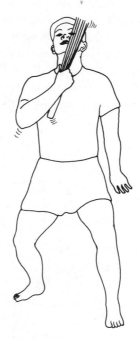

FIGURE 4-20
Gently tapping the head and jaw

7. Left and Right Inside Elbows

NOTE: The insides of the elbows should be hit separately before Hitting the lines of the arms, and then again afterwards to conclude the exercise. First inhale, pack, and pull up the undertrunk while contracting the muscles around the left inner elbow. Concentrate on this area, and hit the inside of the joint three times. (Figure 4-21) Exhale, relax, and absorb the Chi. Hit the inside joint of the right arm in the same manner. The back of each knee joint should also be hit this way before starting the leg sequences.

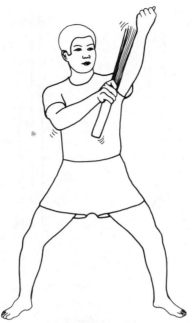

FIGURE 4-21
Hitting the left and right inside elbows

There are six meridians on the arms: the three inside lines of the middle finger, the thumb, and the pinky, and the outside lines of the index finger, the fourth finger, and the pinky. If you find that you have little time to hit all six lines, then only hit the two inside lines of the middle finger and the thumb, and the two outside lines of the pinky and the back of the hand. (These four lines are used in the chapter Summary.) Always lower the arm to reach the outside meridian associated with the small finger. See Figure 4-22 for the six meridians of the arms.

8. Inside Elbow—Middle Finger Line

Extend your left arm above the level of your shoulders with the palm facing up. Hit the inside of the left elbow three more times, then continue Hitting along the center of the arm to the inside wrist, through the palm, to the tip of the middle finger. (Figure 4-23) Return using the same route, traversing the inner elbow, to reach the shoulder at the front of the collarbone. Rest, absorb the energy, then move to the next line.

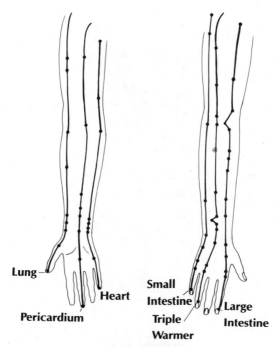

Lung

Heart

Pericardium

Small Intestine

Triple Warmer

Large Intestine

FIGURE 4-22
The six meridians of the arms

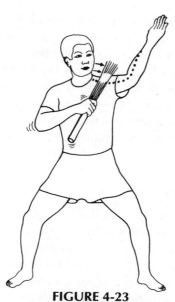

FIGURE 4-23
Hitting the Middle Finger Line

9. Inside Elbow—Thumb Line

With the arm extended above the shoulder, and the palm facing up, hit three times the point located near the outside part of the inner elbow, slightly to the left of its center, where the radius bone begins. Hit towards the hand from this point, over the upper part of the inner wrist, to the inside tip of the thumb, and then return by the same line to the shoulder at the top of the collarbone, over the clavicle. (Figure 4-24) Rest, absorb the energy, then move to the next line.

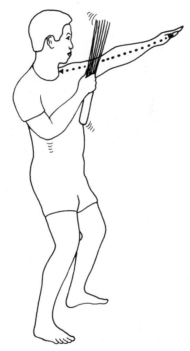

FIGURE 4-24
Hitting the Thumb Line from the shoulder to the thumb

10. Inside Elbow—Pinky Finger Line

With the arm raised above the shoulder and the palm facing up, hit three times the point inside of the inner left elbow, slightly to the right of its center, where the ulna bone begins. Hit towards the hand, over the lower part of the inner left wrist, to the inside tip of the pinky finger. (Figure 4-25) Return by this same line to the shoulder near the chest. Rest, absorb the energy, then move on to the next line.

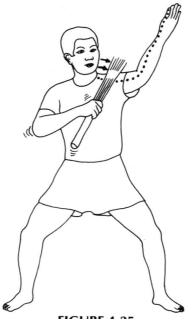

FIGURE 4-25
Inside Pinky Finger Line

11. Outside Elbow—Index Finger Line

With the arm raised above the shoulders, palm face down, and thumb slightly lower than the pinky, hit a point to the right of the outside left elbow three times. From this position the point should appear almost directly between the centers of the inside and the outside of the elbow, on top of the radius bone. Hit towards the back of the hand from this point until you reach the outside tip of the index finger, then return along the same line to the left shoulder. (Figure 4-26) Rest, absorb the energy, then move on to the next line.

12. Outside Elbow—Fourth Finger Line

Lower the arm, extending it beneath the shoulder level with the palm facing down. Turn the wrist so that the thumb is lower than the pinky finger. Bend the left elbow and feel the depression located slightly inward from the tip of the outer elbow, between the tip and the first visible protrusion of the elbow joint. Straighten the left arm and hit this point three times. Continue to hit along this line toward the back of the hand, traversing the outside wrist, over the knuckles, to

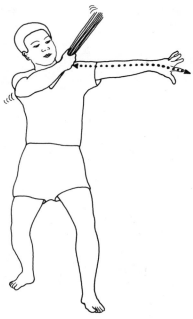

FIGURE 4-26
Outside Index Finger Line

the tip of the fourth finger. (Figure 4-27) Return the Hitting process all the way back up this same line to the top part of the shoulder. Rest, absorb the energy, then move on to the next line.

13. Outside Elbow—Pinky Finger Line

Lower the left arm with the palm directly facing outward, turning the wrist vertically so that the pinky finger is the highest point directly over the thumb, which should point to the floor. Begin Hitting three times the point near the tip of the outside left elbow, continuing the process all the way along the ulna bone, over the outside wrist, to the tip of the pinky finger. (Figure 4-28) Return along the same line to the back of the shoulder by the scapula, near the armpit.

Finish the left arm by again Hitting the center point of the inside elbow three times. The right arm should be hit in the same manner as the left in order to cover the other aspects of the same meridians. Rest, absorb the energy, and then move on to the lines of the right arm. You may hit the left arm and leg together before practicing on the right arm and right leg.

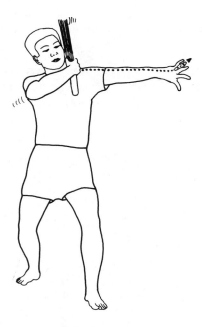

FIGURE 4-27
The Fourth Finger Line

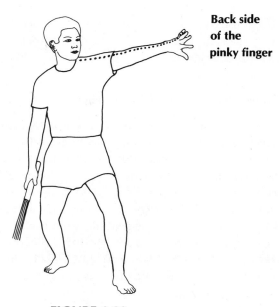

**Back side
of the
pinky finger**

FIGURE 4-28
Hitting the Outside Pinky Line from the shoulder to the fingertip

14. Left and Right Posterior Knee Joints

The six leg meridians are accessed through four Hitting lines—one in back, two on the sides, and one that passes down the middle in front. Start awakening the energy of the legs by Hitting the sacrum three times, since energy tends to concentrate there. Then pack and hit the inside of each knee joint the same way you did the insides of the elbows. (Figure 4-29)

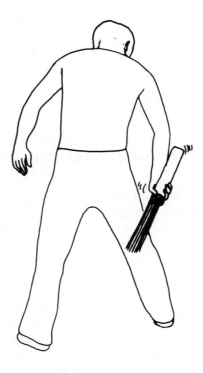

FIGURE 4-29
The Heel Line

15. The Back Side of the Left Leg—Heel Line

Begin by moving your right leg forward and bending it slightly, while the left leg remains straight at a comfortable angle. With the device held in your left hand, hit the back of the left knee three more times, then pack and hit from the left buttocks down to the heel of the

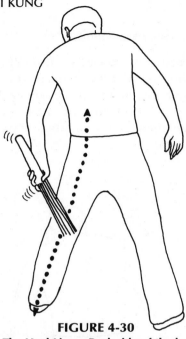

FIGURE 4-30
The Heel Line—Back side of the leg

left foot. (Figure 4-30) Return the process back up along the same line, covering the starting position, to a point on the back three inches directly to the left of the Ming Men. Rest, absorb the energy, then move on to the next line.

16. Outside Left Leg—Small Toe Line

Maintain the stance above, and hit the point left of center on the outside of the left knee three times. Pack and hit the outside of the leg from the hip down to the outer edge of the ankle, ending at the tip of the small toe. (Figure 4-31(a)) Return back up this same route to finish where you began. (Figure 4-31(b)) Rest, absorb the energy, and then move to the next line.

17. Inside Left Leg—Big Toe Line

With your feet parallel, move your left leg one half-step to the side. Men should use the right hand to cover the genitals, pulling them away from the left side. Pack and hit three times the point located on the inner side of the joint, to the right of the knee, between the kneecap and the back of the leg.

From a point near your genitals, which are protected, continue

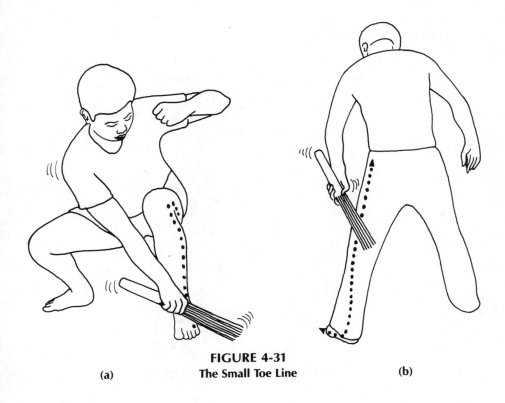

FIGURE 4-31

(a)　　　　　　　　**The Small Toe Line**　　　　　　　　(b)

Packing and Hitting down along the inside of the leg, covering the inside of the ankle completely, to the tip of the big toe. Hit the ankle area three additional times since the spleen, liver, and kidney meridians meet near the ankle on this line. (Avoid Hitting the protrusion of the ankle bone directly.) Return back up this same line to the starting point near the genitals. (Figure 4-32) Rest, absorb the energy, and then move on to the next line.

18. The Front of the Leg—Middle Toe Line

Stand with the left leg forward slightly, and hold the device in the right hand. Hit a point below the center of the left kneecap three times gently. (Hit beneath the kneecap, not directly on it.) Reposition the Hitting device to the point at which the leg meets the body in the middle of the leg, directly between the hip and the sexual center.

Hit down the front of the leg, covering the knee, over the tarsus of the foot, to the tip of the middle toe. (Figure 4-33) Gently hit the area at the top of the foot, in the middle, an additional three times. Return back up this line to end where you started the process. Hit the point at the back of the knee three times to finish the process. Rest, absorb the energy, and then move on to the lines of the right leg.

153

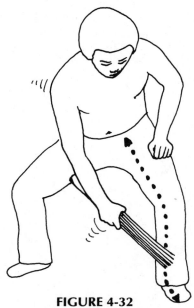

FIGURE 4-32
Hitting the Big Toe Line of the leg

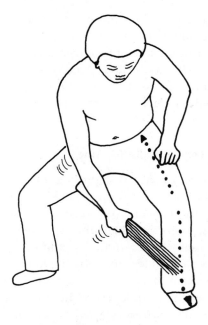

FIGURE 4-33
Hitting the Middle Line of the leg

19. The Sole of the Foot or "Bubbling Spring"

Hitting the bottom of each foot helps to increase the Chi flow and the circulation, returning blood to the heart faster through the veins. It also helps to open a channel for earth energy to be drawn into the body. You may sit on a chair and strike the point illustrated in Figure 4-34 from nine to 36 times. Rest, and absorb the energy.

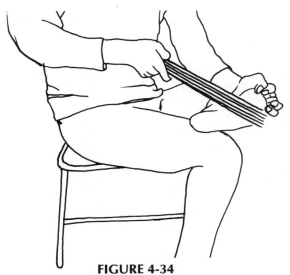

FIGURE 4-34
Hitting the Sole of the Foot ("Bubbling Spring")

F. HITTING WITH RATTAN STICKS

WARNING: THE NECK, RIBS, KNEECAPS, SACRUM, SPINE, AND ALL JOINTS MUST BE CAREFULLY AVOIDED WHEN USING THE RATTAN STICKS. With this in mind, you may apply this procedure to the lines described in the summary after carefully reading the precautions in Section G.

Hitting with Rattan Sticks does not create vibrations within the body as does Hitting with the wire device, but it increases your tolerance for pain and releases tension in the muscles, detoxifies the skin, and enhances lymphocyte production. It also helps the nerves to conduct impulses more effectively while increasing the production of hormones. The Hitting lines for rattan sticks are identical to those used for the other methods, but several areas must be avoided.

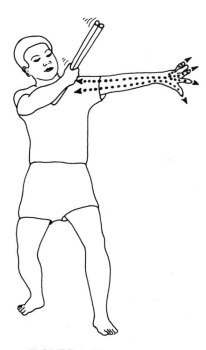

FIGURE 4-35
Hitting the bones of the lower arms with the rattan sticks will toughen them

This practice is usually done immediately after the other Hitting methods. It is important to remember not to use any Packing, and to avoid Hitting the bones. NEVER hit the sacrum or the spinal cord with the rattans. Unlike the other methods, the rattan sticks are used sparsely on the two side lines extending over the kidneys. During this procedure, the scapulae must be rounded and separated by extending the arms as you hit their respective lines. For this reason it is best to have a partner apply the device for you.

Certain areas, such as the shin bones and the ulna and radius bones of the lower arm, can be toughened to improve one's abilities in martial arts or in contact sports. (Figure 4-35) The shins tend to be very sensitive, so the rattan sticks should be applied very lightly from the top of the shins down, and then back up again. (Figure 4-36) As a rule, however, it is best to hit where there are not too many bones. (Figure 4-37) You should also be especially careful to avoid the face, neck, spine, and kneecaps. The point here is to absorb the shock of wood upon skin, thereby detoxifying the skin and strengthening the nerves while the pain is transformed into energy.

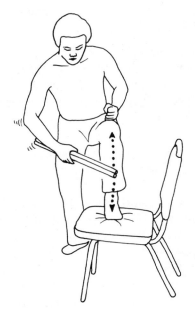

FIGURE 4-36
Carefully Hitting the shins with the Rattan Sticks

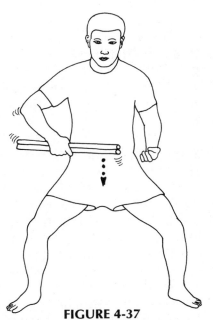

FIGURE 4-37
Hitting below the navel with the Rattan Sticks

G. PRECAUTIONS

WARNING: NEVER APPLY ANY HITTING DEVICE TO AN AREA THAT HAS BEEN BRUISED OR RECENTLY SCARRED IN ANY WAY. THIS WILL ONLY INCREASE THE PAIN AND INHIBIT THE HEALING PROCESS. ALSO AVOID HITTING ANY SORES OR OPEN WOUNDS THAT CAN BE-COME INFECTED OR BLEED AS A RESULT OF THIS PRACTICE.

1. If you have psychological or physical illnesses, or any sexually related problems, consult a doctor or psychologist before attempting this practice.

2. If the Microcosmic Orbit has not been opened, you cannot experience Hitting safely. To avoid severe discomfort and possible damage to your system, be certain that you have a clear flow of internal energy. When Packing is used with Hitting, Chi pressure is increased to the point where energy flows up to the head in quantities greater than the brain can safely handle. A channel must therefore be opened for this energy to travel down from the head to the navel. Be sure that the Microcosmic Orbit is open in order to avoid serious consequences.

3. When Hitting remove all watches, pens, and jewelry that will obstruct your practice, and put them in a safe place.

4. If you are weak or in poor health, you should not use Hitting with Packing because the rush of energy that is produced can be over-whelming to your internal system. Practice Hitting to Detoxify—without Packing—until your health improves.

NOTE: People with high blood pressure, heart disease, or blood clots should refrain from Packing altogether. A physician must be consulted before attempting any form of the Hitting practice in this case.

5. Always use a Hitting technique with the wire device or the long bean bag immediately after the Sexual Energy Massage or Chi Weight Lifting. This is required to help the body assimilate the energy before too much of it rushes to the head with potentially dangerous results.

6. Always try to relax the upper part of the body while practicing. If there is tension in the muscles of the chest, the heart and lungs may become congested with Chi and overheat. If any difficulties occur, such as chest pain, reduce or stop your practice until you are comfortable.

7. Although the sacrum is lightly tapped in detoxifying, do not in any way hit the spinal cord.

8. When Hitting around the neck or the head, clench your teeth,

and place your tongue up against the roof of your mouth to avoid damaging your teeth or biting your tongue.

9. Do not practice Hitting on a full stomach, and do not eat immediately after Hitting. Wait at least two hours after a moderate meal before practicing. Also, it is best to empty the bladder and bowels before a practice session; otherwise large amounts of Chi may be passed out of the body.

10. It is important to remember not to take a shower or bath for at least an hour after you have practiced Hitting, especially if you sweat. Water can wash away external energy, thereby reducing some of the energy you are trying to store. Shower before practicing.

11. Even if you are in good health, if you feel just a little out of sorts, or weak, do not practice Hitting or any exercise that requires Hitting. If you decide to practice at such times, hit only your arms, legs, and back very lightly. Wait at least a day or two, or until you again feel alert and vigorous, before striking areas where the impact might reach vital organs.

12. Make sure that you get sufficient rest after Hitting; the detoxification may exhaust you. Drink plenty of pure water to help the cleansing process.

13. Burp freely during practice; your body will feel the need to eliminate the trapped toxins and gases that are released from within.

H. SUMMARY OF HITTING

The following summary can be used with or without Packing for all applications. The areas to avoid with the rattan sticks are indicated.

1. The Abdomen

a. Preliminary Hitting: To stimulate energies and detoxify, hit three times the Lower Tan Tien (below the navel), the Ming Men (opposite the navel on the spine), the inside of both elbows, and the backs of both knees. Remember to hit the inside elbows three times before and after practicing on the lines of the arms. Also hit the backs of the knees before and after Hitting the legs.

b. Hit from the navel down to the pubic bone, and then back up to the sternum.

c. Hit down a parallel line from a point one and a half inches to the left of the navel, and then back up to beneath the ribs.

d. Hit down a parallel line from a point three inches to the left of the navel, and then back up to the ribs.

e. Apply the same procedures to lines running parallel on the right side of the abdomen at one and a half inches and three inches respectively.

2. The Rib Cage

Do not use rattan sticks to hit the rib cage.

a. Apply the wire device to the ribs from the sternum extending outward horizontally, starting at the base of the rib cage, Hitting towards the left side, then repositioning the device higher at the sternum for each rib. Apply the same procedures to the right side of the chest. (Always hold the device at an angle, pointing out to the side.)

b. Gently tap the sternum to stimulate the thymus, then extend the Hitting lines upward and out to both sides of the collarbone.

3. The Lines of the Back

Avoid the sacrum and spine when Hitting with the rattan sticks.

Sink in the chest as you round out both scapulae by extending your arms. Using the wire device, lightly hit from the left kidney up to the left side of the neck at the base of the skull, and then back down. Change the hand holding the device if necessary. Always clench the teeth. Apply the same procedures to the right side.

4. Left and Right Sides of the Body

Raise your left arm and hit downward from the floating ribs to the left hip. Then hit back up to the armpit, returning finally to the floating ribs. Repeat the same procedure on the right side.

5. The Head and Jaw

Do not apply the rattan sticks to the head and jaw.

Gently tap with the wire device from the forehead around the skull, avoiding the crown. Use the device cautiously around the lower jaw. Remember to clench the teeth whenever you hit the neck, head, or jaw.

6. The Lines of the Arms

Avoid Hitting wrists, knuckles, and elbows with the rattan sticks.

Although there are six meridians in each arm and leg, there are four Hitting lines commonly used to access them from the surface of each limb. Use these four lines when you do not have time to hit all six.

NOTE: Three of the following Hitting lines require that either arm be held up higher than its shoulder as it is hit. Only the Pinky Line requires that the arm be held down.

a. THE MIDDLE FINGER LINE

Raise the left arm, palm up, fingers extended. Hit the inside of the elbow three times, then continue Hitting as you move the striker toward the middle finger on the palm side. Use the same process as you return toward the shoulder, up to the base of the neck. End by Hitting the inner elbow three more times.

b. THE THUMB LINE

Raise the left arm, thumb side up, and hit from the top of the inner elbow—close to the outside of the arm—to the end of the thumb, and then back towards the shoulder until you reach the neck line.

c. THE BACK OF THE HAND

Raise the left arm, palm down, and hit from the side of the elbow down to the tip of the middle finger, and then back to the shoulder once again.

d. THE PINKY LINE

Lower your left arm in front of you, thumb pointing down, palm facing out vertically so that the small finger is on top. Hit from the base of the elbow to the tip of the pinky finger, and then back up to the posterior of the collarbone.

You may apply the device to the other arm now, or you may hit the lines of the left leg before using these procedures on the right arm and leg.

7. The Lines of the Legs

Avoid kneecaps, toes, and ankle bones when Hitting with the rattan sticks.

a. THE MIDDLE LINE

Hit from the top of the left leg—where it joins the body in front—down to the tips of the toes, and then back up to the starting point.

b. THE BIG TOE LINE

Men should cover the genital area. Hit the inner leg from the inner thigh down to the inside of the big toe, and then back up to the starting point.

c. THE SMALL TOE LINE

Hit the outer left leg from the hip joint down to the small toe, and then back up to the starting point.

d. THE BACKS OF THE LEGS

Hit from the buttocks to the heel of the left foot, emphasizing the back of the knee, then return up this route to the starting point. Hit the back of the knee three more times to finish the left leg. You may now reposition the Hitting device and begin the process on the same four lines of the right leg, or on the right arm and leg together.

8. The Soles of the Feet ("Bubbling Spring")

You may sit in a chair to hit the soles of the feet. Hit each from nine to 36 times, rest, and absorb the energy.

Chapter Five

CHI WEIGHT LIFTING

The ancient Taoist masters discovered that the genitals were connected to the organs and glands in an area of the perineum called the "Chi Muscle," which encompasses the anal, perineal, and pubic-coccygeal muscles. (Figure 5-1) With this knowledge they developed the Healing Love techniques, using the Chi Muscle to create an upward flow of sexual energy into the higher centers of the body. They eventually learned to increase this Chi flow by developing the "fasciae," which are connective tissues engaged by the organs and glands to lift weights externally anchored to the genitals in the Chi Weight Lifting practice. (Figure 5-2) The beneficial aspects of strengthening the internal system through the fasciae became an integral part of Bone Marrow Nei Kung.

Originally, men accomplished Chi Weight Lifting by placing stones in a basket and hanging the basket from their groins. Today, male and female Taoists use light weights to draw a special formula of sexual energy from the genitals upward into the body. This sexual energy, or Ching Chi, is combined with external energy and compressed into the skeletal structure through the methods described in this book. As sexual energy transforms into life-force energy, Chi Weight Lifting en-

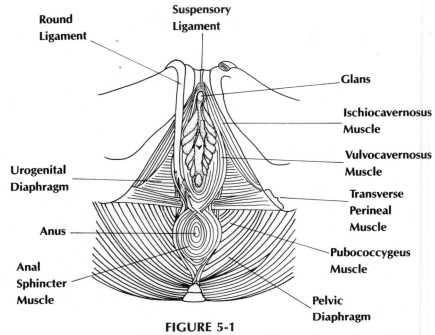

Round Ligament

Suspensory Ligament

Glans

Ischiocavernosus Muscle

Vulvocavernosus Muscle

Urogenital Diaphragm

Transverse Perineal Muscle

Anus

Pubococcygeus Muscle

Anal Sphincter Muscle

Pelvic Diaphragm

FIGURE 5-1

The Chi Muscle includes the urogenital diaphragm, the pelvic diaphragm, the anal sphincter muscle, and the pubococcygeus (PC) muscle

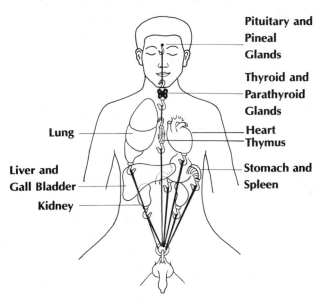

Pituitary and Pineal Glands

Thyroid and Parathyroid Glands

Lung

Heart Thymus

Liver and Gall Bladder

Stomach and Spleen

Kidney

FIGURE 5-2

The sexual organs are joined to all of the organs, glands, tendons, and muscles

hances the life-force of the men and women who practice it. The genitals are replenished by the rejuvenated organs and glands as the transformed energy returns through the Microcosmic Orbit.

A. APPLICATIONS FOR CHI WEIGHT LIFTING

1. Strengthening the Fasciae Network

An upward counterforce is created by the internal organs and glands to resist the weight placed upon the genitals. This force is strengthened by the Chi released from the sexual center as the internal system engages the fasciae to pull up against the weight. The fasciae, therefore, contribute greatly to the distribution of energy. They also serve as the connection between the genitalia and the pelvic and urogenital diaphragms. When this connection is loose, the Chi Muscle and the diaphragms allow the organs to drop their weight onto the perineum, thereby reducing the Chi pressure. When the connection is kept strong, the organs and glands are held in place, and the Chi pressure is maintained.

2. Chi Weight Lifting for Powerful Urogenital and Pelvic Diaphragms

The human body has many diaphragms holding the internal organs and glands in place, such as the thoracic, pelvic, and urogenital diaphragms. During Chi Weight Lifting these contribute greatly to the upward counterforce deployed against the downward pull of the weights anchored to the genitals. (Figure 5-3) The pelvic and urogenital diaphragms, considered the floor of the organs, and the Chi Muscle, are all strengthened by this practice which helps to prevent any loss of energy through them. Their increased strength also helps to alleviate the protruding abdomen caused by organs stacking up on the pelvic area. (Figure 5-4)

Chi Weight Lifting is credited with many other benefits related to the improved functioning of the diaphragms, such as the lifting of dropped kidneys. Furthermore, the practice helps to seal the openings of the anus and sex organ to prevent the leakage of Chi. Taoists believe that this helps to redirect the spirit away from these openings as one prepares to finally leave the body. The upward flow of energy that is developed through Taoist practices will point toward the crown as the proper exit for the spirit to use at the end of life.

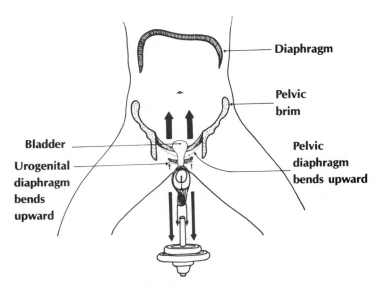

FIGURE 5-3
The pelvic and urogenital diaphragms provide counterforce to the weights

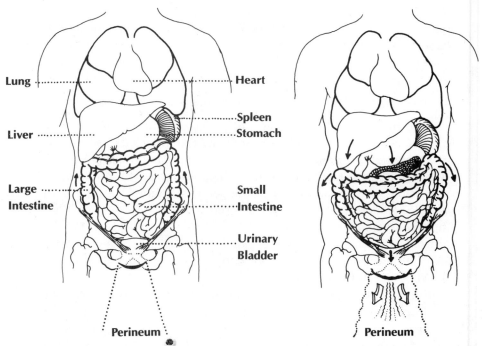

The vital organs are stacked upon the perineum. A strong perineum prevents the organs from sagging down

A weak perineum allows Chi to leak out as the internal organs sag, dropping their weight upon each other

FIGURE 5-4

3. Sexual Hormones Delay the Aging Process

The release of sexual hormones stimulates the pituitary gland to prevent the production of an aging hormone. It has been proposed that one function of this gland may be to measure the growth of mutated reproductive cells. Scientific studies have found some evidence that the aging hormone is released when these mutations are allowed to increase beyond a certain level. Theoretically, their growth should be impeded by a healthy reserve of sexual hormones. Otherwise, upon sensing the reduced presence of Ching Chi within the body, the pituitary gland can cause a premature death by producing the aging hormone. It is therefore wise to maintain sexual energy and hormones through the Taoist practices.

4. Sexual Hormone Stimulation of the Brain

The right side of the brain is also influenced by the sexual hormones to promote the healing and rejuvenation of the body. Since Ching Chi revitalizes the internal system and regrows the bone marrow, hormonal stimulation of the brain greatly enhances these processes. This effect also serves Taoist spiritual work because practitioners find it to be an invigorating experience on all levels. The health of the body and the mind directly affects the spirit.

B. EQUIPMENT AND EXTERNAL PREPARATIONS

1. The Cloth for the Massage and Lifting the Weight

Men and women use a silk cloth for the Sexual Energy Massage techniques to increase the flow of Chi and blood in their sexual centers. Silk works well because it develops considerable static energy when rubbed. This is important for the stimulation of Chi in the sexual organs, perineum and sacrum. Women also use the cloth to massage their breasts. Men use the cloth after the massage techniques to lift the weight from a special holding apparatus.

MEN: Two sizes of cloth can be used to lift the weight, depending on the method chosen for practice. The smaller cloth, which is used for lifting the weight from a table or chair, should measure approximately three and one-half by eight inches. If you choose to lift the weight from the floor, the length of the cloth can vary according to the length of your legs. When the cloth has been cut to size, you can sew the edges to prevent unraveling and to avoid abrasions of the skin.

2. Equipment for Men and Women

a. EQUIPMENT FOR MEN

Men require a special device by which the weight can be held to the cloth. (Figure 5-5) Cut a ten inch length of galvanized pipe for an apparatus to be used from the floor. Cut an eight inch length for an apparatus to be used from a chair. (Either size is adaptable to either method if necessary.) Drill a one-quarter inch hole through the pipe one-half inch from either end.

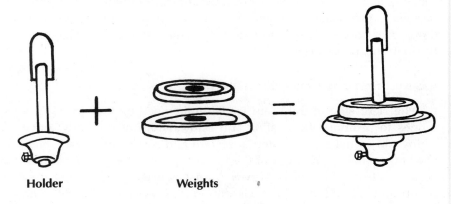

Holder   Weights

FIGURE 5-5
Weight lifting device for men

Secure a piece of chain two links long to the pipe with a one-quarter inch bolt inserted through the hole and fastened by a nut and washer at its end. At the end of the chain, a heavy ring one and a half inches in diameter is attached. Several types of clamps may be used on the opposite end of the pipe to hold the weights. After the silk cloth has been tied gently, but firmly, around the groin, it can then be attached to the ring in order to lift the entire weight-holding apparatus.

Some men can begin Chi Weight Lifting with a two and one-half pound weight; however, it is safer to start with the apparatus alone, or with one or two weight clamps attached to it. (These are used in standard barbell sets.) If you use two weight clamps, their weight should equal one pound, plus the weight of the apparatus itself. Some stores that carry sporting equipment sell one and a half pound weights. Add on more weight gradually, but only as much as you feel comfortable with. Do not advance to higher weights unless you can lift the current weight easily for one minute.

b. EQUIPMENT FOR WOMEN

Women require a special egg drilled lengthwise for the insertion of a string which holds the weight. (See Chapter Three.) The egg is inserted into the vagina, large end first, with the string tied to the weight. Squatting may make it easier to insert the egg as the weight rests on the floor. The weight is then lifted and swung like a pendulum. Jade eggs are recommended. Obsidian eggs can also be drilled to accommodate the string, but they may require a diamond drill bit.

It is recommended that all eggs be drilled, even if weights are not used, because the string can help in removing the egg. Jade eggs are preferable because they are sturdy, smooth, and non-porous. You may also find that jade eggs are far less expensive. Wooden eggs, or any eggs with painted or chemical finishes should be avoided. Prior to Chi Weight Lifting, training with the egg should begin with the techniques explained in Chapter Three. The egg exercise must first be mastered without any weight.

Women can begin Chi Weight Lifting with a one-half pound weight, gradually adding one-half pound at a time. A string can be tied to the men's weight lifting apparatus, first using the bar alone as a trial weight. (Figure 5-6) (Light weights are also available that can be tied

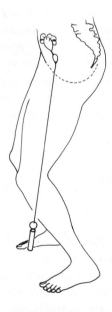

FIGURE 5-6
Women can begin lifting by using the lifting apparatus alone

directly onto the string without the bar.) Later, try using the men's apparatus with one or two weight clamps, which are used in standard barbell sets. Finally, when you are ready, try lifting the apparatus with a weight held on by one of the clamps. It is better to lift lighter weights for longer periods than heavier weights for shorter periods. Never exceed one minute.

3. Preparations for Men and Women

After learning one of the tying methods, or how to use the egg, test yourself with the weight-holding apparatus before you add any weights to it. If it feels light to you, begin adding the weight clamps. Later, you may start adding standard weights. When you are ready, you can increase the weight until a maximum of two and a half pounds is reached. DO NOT ATTEMPT TO EXCEED THIS LEVEL ON THE FIRST DAY. Instead, try to sustain the weight for longer periods— but less than a minute—to release more energy.

Swinging the weight will gently increase the pressure. This is preferable to increasing the weights too fast, or to lifting them too long. Each swing back and forth can be counted as one second. Practice at each level until you can easily lift the weight for up to 60 seconds. Men must be careful not to cut off the circulation to the testicles. Lifting for more than a minute can impede circulation.

The room in which you practice should be quiet and well ventilated, but not cold. Keep a hard chair available for your meditation and as a place to rest the weight, unless you lift from the floor. As suggested earlier, the best time for these exercises is the morning after you shower and relieve your bladder and bowels. If you can, face the sun as you practice in the early morning hours, but never look directly into it at any time.

C. STARTING THE PRACTICE

1. When to Start

MEN: In determining when it is safe to begin Chi Weight Lifting, consider the condition of your testicles and scrotum. If the scrotum is very loose and hanging weakly, and the testicles feel weak, practice only the massage techniques. Do not practice Chi Weight Lifting. If the testicles are too tight and close to the body, none of the tying methods will work. Massage the testicles until they loosen.

The optimum condition for weight lifting is when the testicles are slightly loose, but firm. The strength of the testicles can be felt internally rather than with the fingers. In other words, when they are massaged their resilience and ability to withstand the massage without pain will indicate their condition. A slight pain from the first massage may be the result of a beginner's apprehensions. Do not begin to practice weight lifting until you are comfortable emotionally as well as physically.

WOMEN: There is less danger for women in the Chi Weight Lifting practice. You are ready when, after massaging the breasts and genitals, the vagina is moist with secretions. If not enough moisture is present, prepare the vagina with a natural lubricating cream. Women can feel reasonably safe with these practices—provided that the egg and string are kept sanitary—because the weights can be easily released if they prove too heavy to lift.

2. Weight Lifting Goals

The Healing Tao does not recommend anyone try to lift over ten pounds without supervision. On the basis of this book, ten pounds should be considered the absolute maximum goal. Women may find that their lifting capabilities are slightly different because they have no way to anchor the weight and are therefore more dependent upon internal power. It is certainly no shame for men and women to lift less than the one or two pounds recommended for beginners. If you choose to lift beyond five pounds, exercise more than the usual caution.

WARNING: Lifting heavier weights without supervision is both foolish and contrary to the recommendations of this book. In systems where excessive weights are used for practice, broken veins or blood clots have occurred in some overzealous men, resulting in serious injury. (There are no statistics available concerning possible deaths that may have occurred.) Further instruction in Bone Marrow Nei Kung is necessary for Chi Weight Lifting with heavier weights. Contact the Healing Tao Center for information on advanced instruction.

D. GENITAL MASSAGE AND PREPARATORY EXERCISES FOR MEN AND WOMEN

1. The Massage Techniques

Review Chapter Three for the Cloth Massage and Sexual Energy

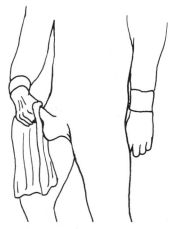

FIGURE 5-7
The Cloth Massage

Massage practices. These stimulate internal energies and prepare the genitals for the role at hand. (Figure 5-7) First, the silk cloth is applied to the sexual center, perineum, and sacrum to activate the Chi. Men should feel the testicles fill with energy as they become firm. Women should feel the breasts enlarge slightly as the vagina becomes moist with secretions. The Sexual Energy Massage techniques should then be used to condition the genitals for Chi Weight Lifting. After the weights are removed, the massage techniques must be repeated to restore the circulation of blood and Chi to the sexual center.

MEN: Although not all six techniques are required, the Sexual Energy Massage must be emphasized by men after the weights have been removed to ensure that the genital area will be clear of any blood coagulation which can lead to blood clots.

2. An Outline of Pre-Chi Weight Lifting Exercises

Review Chapter Three for the practices listed here. Both men and women should specifically review the Power Lock, which is used before the Sexual Energy Massage and again immediately after the weights have been removed. The Kidney and Chi Pressure exercises are included herein.

MEN:
    (a) Increasing Chi Pressure exercise
    (b) Increasing Kidney Pressure
    (c) Power Lock—two or three times up to the crown

    (d) Cloth Massage

    (e) Finger Massage of the Testicles

    (f) Palm Massage of the Testicles

    (g) Ducts Elongation Rubbing

    (h) Stretching the Ducts Gently with Massage

    (i) Stretching the Scrotum and Penis Tendons

    (j) Tapping the Testicles

WOMEN:

    (a) Increasing Chi Pressure exercise

    (b) Increasing Kidney Pressure

    (c) Power Lock—two or three times up to the crown

    (d) Cloth Massage

    (e) Breast Massage

    (f) Massage the Glands with Accumulated Chi

    (g) Massage the Organs with Accumulated Chi

    (h) Massage the Ovaries

    (i) Egg Exercise (optional)

a. INCREASING CHI PRESSURE

Before you initiate the Power Lock exercise, you should be certain that the abdomen is full of Chi. Place the middle finger of each hand about one and one-half inches below the navel. Concentrate on the Lower Tan Tien as you inhale Chi into it, expanding the point with the resulting pressure. Your mental power increases the energy flow to this area. Exhale, and release the pressure. (Figure 5-8) Repeat this exercise up to 81 times.

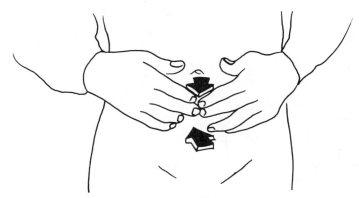

FIGURE 5-8
Inhale and exhale up to 81 times to the lower abdomen to increase Chi pressure. Use the fingers to press in

b. INCREASING KIDNEY PRESSURE

   Stand in a Horse Stance with your feet slightly wider than shoulder width. Rub your hands together until they are warm, and then apply their warmth to the kidneys by placing your energized palms on them from the back. (Figure 5-9 (a) and (b)) Bend your upper body forward slightly as you inhale, and pull up the left and right sides of the anus as you draw Chi up to the kidneys. (Figure 5-9(c)) Exhale, and deflate the kidneys. Follow this sequence up to 36 times, and finish by warming the hands and again placing them on the kidneys.

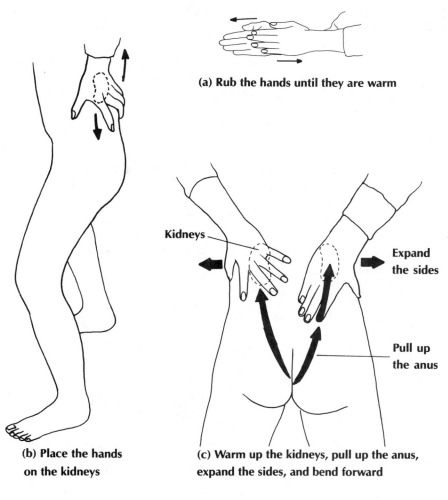

(a) Rub the hands until they are warm

Kidneys

Expand the sides

Pull up the anus

(b) Place the hands on the kidneys

(c) Warm up the kidneys, pull up the anus, expand the sides, and bend forward

FIGURE 5-9
Increasing kidney pressure

E. CHI WEIGHT LIFTING IN DETAIL

WARNING: DO NOT ATTEMPT CHI WEIGHT LIFTING WITHOUT STUDYING THE PRECAUTIONS IN SECTION F.

Students are expected to receive instruction before attempting Chi Weight Lifting; however, the following detailed synopsis will clarify this practice for novices. Students are not expected to remember every detail. In advanced practice, the steps which follow are combined into a very brief exercise. Although the summary is concise enough to be used as a practice guide for trained practitioners, ALL PRACTITIONERS ARE ADVISED TO FIRST READ THE DETAILS.

1. Attaching the Weight—MEN

a. THE POSITION OF THE WEIGHTS

Chi Weight Lifting can be initiated from either a kneeling or standing position. (Figure 5-10) If you cannot kneel, set the weight on a chair

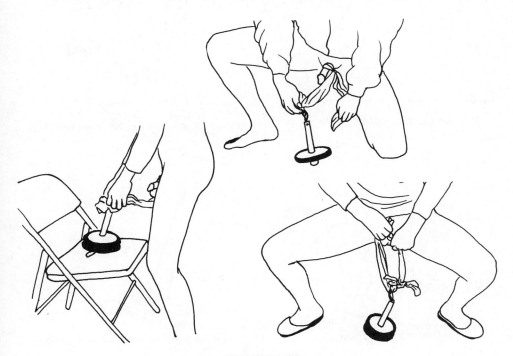

FIGURE 5-10
Chi Weight Lifting can be initiated from either a kneeling or a standing position

175

in front of you. It may be necessary to relieve the pressure of the weights quickly at times, particularly if they are too heavy and the knot beneath the testicles is tight. For this reason, keep the weight close to a place where it can be quickly removed. Consider tying one end of the cloth to the ring while leaving the other end in a loop—folded beneath the knot—so that the knot will undo itself if that end is pulled.

b. A STANDARD METHOD OF TYING THE CLOTH

WARNING: DO NOT TIE THE CLOTH AROUND THE TESTICLES ALONE.

(1) Fold the cloth lengthwise several times to a width of about one inch. (Figure 5-11) This creates a thick padding.

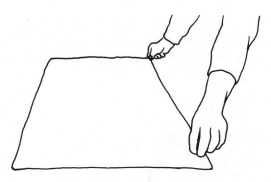

(a) Lay the cloth flat

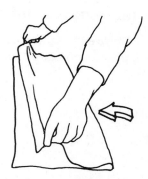

(b) Fold it in half with the edges matched

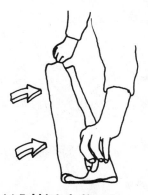

(c) Fold it in half again

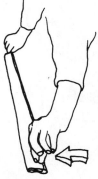

(d) Fold it again into a thick strip of padding

FIGURE 5-11
Folding the cloth

(2) Hold the cloth beneath the perineum, and bring it up behind the testicles. Be sure that the edge of the cloth is folded away from the skin so that it does not cut into the groin.

(3) Wrap both ends of the cloth upward around the penis and testicles, and secure the cloth at the surface of the penis base by tying a knot.

NOTE: If you prefer, you can place the cloth on top of the penis and tie the knot beneath the testicles. In either case, the knot must eventually be positioned at the perineum. (Figure 5-12(a), (b) and (c))

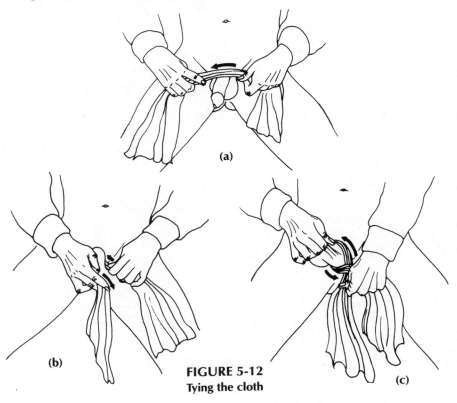

(a)

(b)

FIGURE 5-12
Tying the cloth

(c)

(4) Move the knot behind the testicles and beneath the perineum. The ends of cloth should hang to the floor. Before tightening the knot, you can use one end to create a loop between the knot and the groin so that the cloth and apparatus can be quickly removed.

(5) Contract the muscles of the undertrunk and tighten the knot. The penis and testicles should bulge slightly from the pressure to

insure against slippage. DO NOT CUT OFF THE CIRCULATION TO THE TESTICLES.

(6) Tie one end of the cloth to the weight that you have placed on the floor, or on a chair. (Figure 5-12(d), (e) and (f)) If the weight is on the floor, tie the cloth to it from a kneeling position.

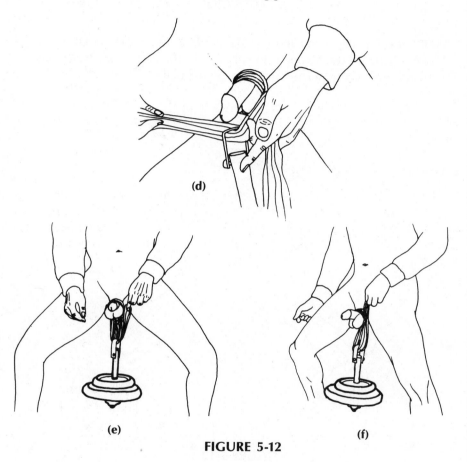

(d)

(e)   (f)

FIGURE 5-12

(7) To remove the weight at the end of practice, kneel in front of the chair—or near the floor—and untie the cloth attached to the holding apparatus, then remove the cloth from the groin.

2. Attaching the Weight—WOMEN:

NOTE: The Internal Egg Exercise described in Chapter Three can be used as a preparation for Chi Weight Lifting. During the actual lifting of weights, however, the egg is held deep inside the vaginal canal. Do not move it up and down, and do not release it.

a. TYING THE STRING TO THE WEIGHT

After the string has been passed through the egg and secured with a knot at the egg's large end, tie the weight to the string. The weight can also be placed inside a bag or container attached to the string. The weight holder prescribed for men can also be used, first without any weight, and then with the gradual addition of the holding clamp and the weight. Either place a chair in front of you and rest the weight on it, or place the weight on the floor and squat down to facilitate the egg's insertion. (Remember to hold the weight with your fingers as you stand up.)

b. INSERTING THE EGG

After you have massaged your breasts and vaginal areas in the pre-scribed manner, kneel down near where the weight is resting, and insert the egg into the vagina, large end first. (Use a lubricant if neces-sary.) Close the vagina, contracting the muscles around the egg to hold it. (Figure 5-13)

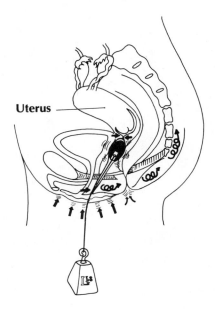

Uterus

FIGURE 5-13
Vaginal Weight Lifting

3. Testing and Lifting the Weight—MEN and WOMEN

(1) Slowly stand up, holding the cloth or the weight in your hand, and assume a weight lifting stance. (Keep the feet parallel at about shoulder width, and bend the knees slightly.) By using your index and middle fingers to test the weight, you can sense whether or not it is too heavy.

(2) Inhale a sip of air, and pull up the anus, perineum, and genitals. Inhale again, and pull up both sides of the anus as you draw Chi into the left and right kidneys respectively.

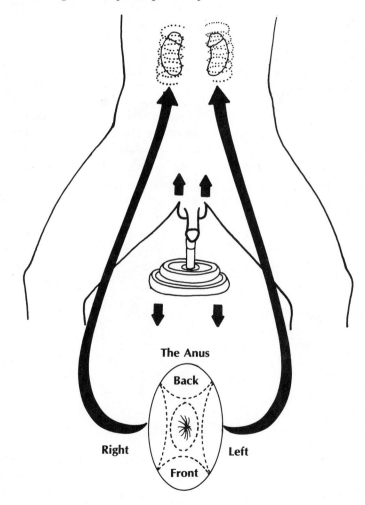

FIGURE 5-14
When you feel the pull of the weight, inhale and pull up the right, left, front, and back parts of the anus. Wrap the Chi around the kidneys

(3) Press the tongue firmly up to the roof of your mouth to increase your internal power. Increasing pressure on this connection will accelerate the upward force of the Chi.

(4) Then, slowly release the cloth or the string from your fingers. You are now sustaining the weight from the sexual organ, and you should begin to pull against it using internal strength, particularly from the kidneys.

(5) With the fingers of one hand nearby, feel the pull of the weight, and determine whether or not your genitals can sustain it. Men in particular should be certain that they are reasonably comfortable.

(6) Inhale, pull up the right, left, front and back sides of the anus, and wrap the energy around the kidneys. (Figure 5-14)

(7) Gently swing the weight, drawing the energy up to the coccyx, and then to the sacrum. You can practice up to the sacrum for the first few weeks. When you feel more energy, you can gradually move it up the spine to T-11, C-7, the Jade Pillow, and all the way to the crown. When you are ready to store the energy, press your tongue to the palate, and bring the energy down to the navel, completing the Microcosmic Orbit.

NOTE: Remember that in advanced practice, a separate round is used to lift the same weight from the internal organs and glands. Rather than remove the weight, you may hold it as you rest between rounds.

(8) To finish the practice, kneel as you place the weight on the chair again, or the floor, and remove the egg and weight holding apparatus. Men should untie the cloth after the apparatus has been removed. The Power Lock should be practiced immediately afterward.

a. SWINGING THE WEIGHT

Swinging the weight gives the practitioner control over the amount of pressure on the groin, which is why lighter weights are recommended. The Chi from the fascial connection between the perineum and the kidneys is used to pull the weight. In the beginning, swing the weights gently as you determine the amount of pressure that is comfortable for you.

Inhale as you contract the anus and perineum. Swing the attached weight from 36 to 49 times. Synchronize your breathing with each swing. Inhale as the weight swings forward, and exhale as it swings backward. (Figure 5-15) Pull up against the weight internally with each forward swing, and draw the energy up to the coccyx, the sacrum,

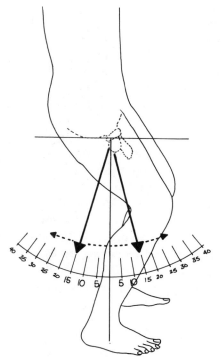

FIGURE 5-15
Swing the weight at an angle between 15 and 30 degrees

and, eventually all the way through the Microcosmic Orbit. (Figure 5-16) Each completed swing back and forth should approximate one second.

After a week, try to swing the weight for 60 counts. More pressure results from the counter-force exerted by the Chi Muscle when heavier weights are swung, but it is wiser to increase this pressure with lighter weights by adding more power to each swing. The lighter weights should be used to their maximum potential, thereby strengthening the Chi Muscle and producing more hormones.

b. FINISH WITH THE POWER LOCK AND MASSAGE TECHNIQUES

Practice the Power Lock for at least two or three rounds after releasing the weight. Then apply the Cloth Massage and the Sexual Energy Massage techniques. Rest, and practice the Microcosmic Orbit Meditation to circulate the tremendous energy you have generated, finally collecting it in the navel.

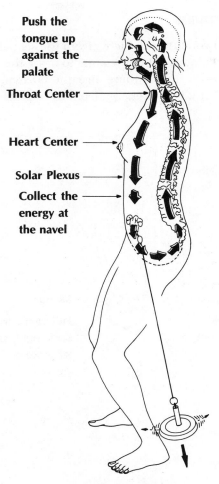

Push the tongue up against the palate

Throat Center

Heart Center

Solar Plexus

Collect the energy at the navel

FIGURE 5-16
Circulate the Chi all the way around the Microcosmic orbit and collect the energy at the navel

4. Lifting Weights from the Microcosmic Orbit: MEN and WOMEN

After you have practiced for two to four weeks, and feel comfortable with Chi Weight Lifting, begin to lift the weight from the stations of the Microcosmic Orbit. As you bring the Chi up into the sacrum and higher centers, use this energy to pull the weight from each station. Take your time, and don't rush. Each point can take one or two weeks before you feel the flow of the Microcosmic Orbit working as part of the counterforce.

a. STEP BY STEP PROCEDURES

(1) Sacrum: When you lift the weights from the sexual organs, pull up the front, back, right and left of the anus to bring the energy up to the sacrum. (Figure 5-17) Hold it there. Breathe normally, and gently swing the weights. Feel a line of energy from the sexual center up to the sacrum.

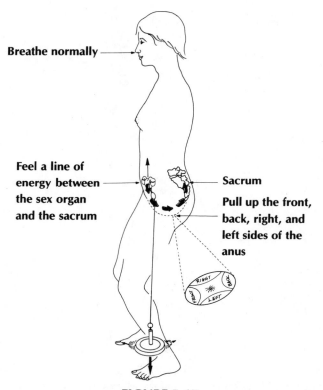

Breathe normally

Feel a line of energy between the sex organ and the sacrum

Sacrum

Pull up the front, back, right, and left sides of the anus

FIGURE 5-17
Swing the weight, pull up the anus at the front, back, right, and left sides, and feel a line of energy between the sex organ and the sacrum

(2) Door of Life: Once you feel the Chi in the sacrum, bring it to the Door of Life on the spine, opposite the navel. (Figure 5- 18) Hold the Chi there, and continue to swing the weights. Every time you swing, pull up more.

(3) T-11 Point: From the Door of Life, bring the energy up to T-11 on the spine, opposite the solar plexus. (Figure 5-19) Feel the line of energy as it moves up to T-11.

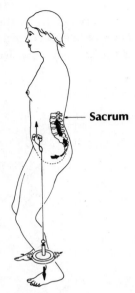

FIGURE 5-18
From the sacrum bring the Chi to the Door of Life (Ming Men)

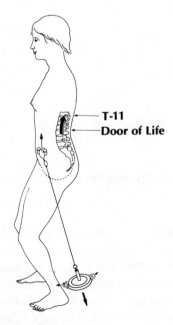

FIGURE 5-19
From the Door of Life bring the energy up to T-11

(4) C-7 Point: Pull the energy from the sexual center, passing it through the sacrum, Door of Life, T-11, and up to C-7 at the base of the neck. (Figure 5-20) Feel the line of energy from the sexual organs up to C-7.

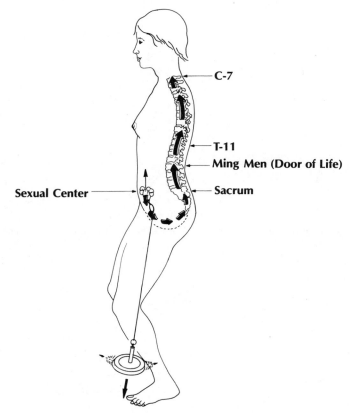

FIGURE 5-20
Pull the energy from the sexual center all the way up to C-7

(5) Base of the Skull: Next draw the Chi through the sacrum, Door of Life, T-11, and C-7, and up to the base of the skull. (Figure 5-21) Feel the line of Chi flow from the sexual organs up to the base of the skull.

(6) Crown Point and the Pineal Gland: Draw the Chi up to the crown point where the pineal gland is located. (Figure 5-22) Remember that the sexual glands are closely related to the pineal and pituitary glands. You may feel this connection as these glands are stimulated.

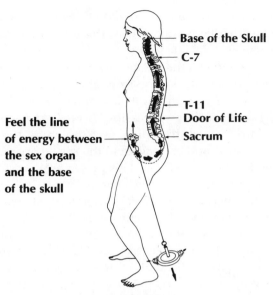

Base of the Skull
C-7

T-11
Door of Life
Sacrum

Feel the line
of energy between
the sex organ
and the base
of the skull

FIGURE 5-21
Pull the Energy from the sex organ all the way up to the base of the skull

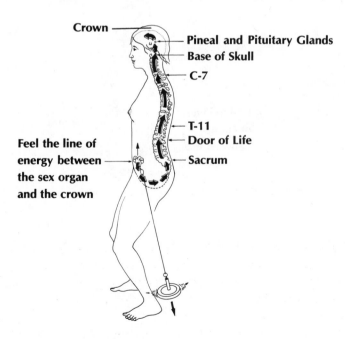

Crown
Pineal and Pituitary Glands
Base of Skull
C-7

T-11
Door of Life
Sacrum

Feel the line of
energy between
the sex organ
and the crown

FIGURE 5-22
Pull the energy from the sex organ all the way to the crown

(7) The Third Eye: Bring the Chi to the "Third Eye" (mid-eyebrow), also called the "Crystal Room," where the pituitary gland is located. (Figure 5-23)

(8) With the tongue on the palate, bring the Chi down to the throat center, the heart center, the solar plexus, and finally down to the navel. (Figure 5-24) The overflow will spill back down to the sexual center.

(9) At this point you have successfully brought the energy from the sexual organs up through the spine, over the top of the head, down the front to the navel, and back again to the sexual organs, circulating it through the Microcosmic Orbit. This process refines and enhances Chi as it moves through the energy centers.

(10) Once the Microcosmic Orbit is open to the flowing sexual energy, all you need do is pull the energy up to the head, and then down to the navel through the tongue. Concentrate on drawing the energy, circulating it in the Microcosmic Orbit, and storing it in the navel. The Chi will flow very quickly through all the centers. You will no longer need to bring it up through the points of the spine one by one.

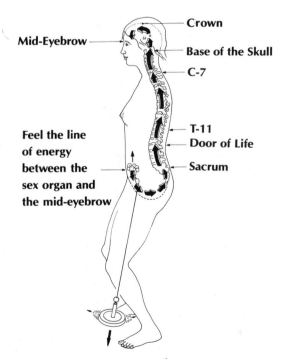

FIGURE 5-23
Pull the energy from the sex organ all the way to the mid-eyebrow

188

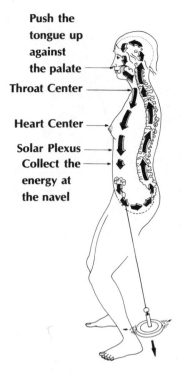

**Push the
tongue up
against
the palate**

Throat Center

Heart Center

**Solar Plexus
Collect the
energy at
the navel**

FIGURE 5-24
**Circulate the Chi all the way around the Microcosmic Orbit and collect the
energy at the navel**

5. ADVANCED CHI WEIGHT LIFTING USING THE INTERNAL ORGANS: MEN AND WOMEN

a. THE KIDNEYS HELP PULL THE WEIGHT

In the beginning stages of Chi Weight Lifting, it is the power of the kidneys that provides real internal counterforce. (Figure 5-25) Once you can feel that power, it becomes easier to tap the force of the other organs to help lift heavier weights. As you begin to increase the weight, start to use the strength of the other organs and glands to increase the upward counterforce. The main secret of internal power is to press the tongue against the roof of the mouth as you direct the force of the organ's energy toward it.

(1) Always begin by pulling the energy up to the head several times to make sure of its flow within the Microcosmic Orbit.

(2) Inhale with small sips, pull up the left side of the anus, and

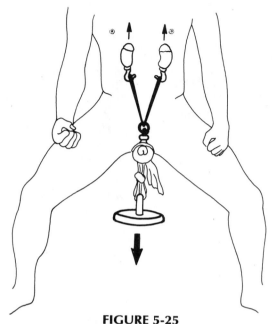

FIGURE 5-25
In the beginning stages of Chi Weight Lifting it is the kidneys that provide the internal counterforce

spiral the energy to the left kidney. Inhale again, pull up the right side of the anus, and spiral the energy into the right kidney. (Figure 5-26) Hold the energy there, and feel the Chi in the kidneys pull up towards the tongue, resisting the weight. Some people report that they can immediately feel the kidneys as they help lift the weight.

(3) Exhale, maintaining the pulling action of the perineum and kidneys, and then breathe normally. With each swing, pull up more on the sexual organs and kidneys. Practice from 36 to 49 swings. Untie the weight, massage the sexual organs, and start Hitting.

b. THE SPLEEN AND LIVER PULL THE WEIGHT

NOTE: Always keep the chest relaxed during these procedures. You can practice lifting from the spleen and liver as a separate exercise, or together as one exercise.

(1) Spleen: Start again on the left side by pulling up the left side of the anus and perineum. Become aware of the spleen situated beneath the left side of the rib cage. Contract the left anus, and pull the Chi up to the spleen and left kidney with one more sip. Wrap the Chi around

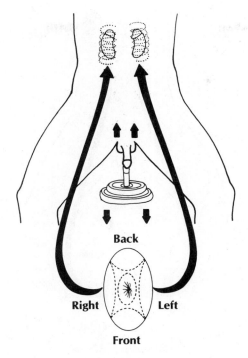

Back

Right   **Left**

Front

FIGURE 5-26
When you feel the pull of the weight, inhale and pull up the right and left side of the anus. Wrap the energy around the kidneys

and into the spleen. (The spleen is located toward the back, slightly above the left kidney and adrenal gland.) Keep the tongue pressed to the roof of your mouth. Then, as you feel its connection to the genitals, pull the spleen energy up towards the tongue. Lift the genitals, thereby lifting the weight.

(2) Liver: Practice the same procedure on the liver, which lies under the right side of the rib cage. Pull up the right side of the anus and perineum. First draw the Chi up to the right kidney. Then become aware of your liver, and pull the Chi up to it twice. Pack and wrap the liver with Chi. Pull the energy toward the back, near the right kidney and adrenal gland. Push the tongue against the roof of your mouth. Then, as you feel its connection to the genitals, draw the liver energy up to the tongue. Pull up the genitals, thereby lifting the weight.

(3) Combine the procedures of the spleen from the left side and the liver from the right side in order to help lift the weight. (Figure 5-27) Pull their combined energies up towards the tongue.

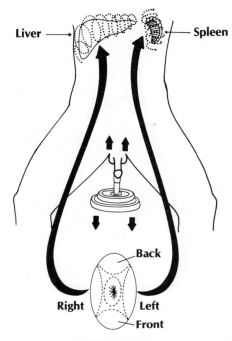

Liver   Spleen

Back

Right   Left

Front

FIGURE 5-27

Inhale and pull up the right side of the anus, directing the energy to the liver.
Inhale and pull up the left side of the anus, directing the energy to the spleen.
Wrap the energy around these organs

c. LIFTING WITH THE LUNGS

Lifting a weight with the lungs is an advanced procedure and is more difficult than lifting with other organs and glands. Before you try to apply Chi Weight Lifting using the lungs, practice pulling energy up to each of the lower organs in succession, drawing the organ energy up toward the tongue. Pull up the Chi of the lower organs until you actually feel each lung contracting. Each step should first be practiced separately. Later, all of the steps can be combined into one practice. The procedure is as follows:

(1) First draw the Chi up from the sexual center through each of the organs and glands in succession. Lift with the kidneys, the spleen, and then with the left lung as the Chi reaches it. Inhale, and expand the upper left stomach near the left rib cage. Inhale again, and pull the stomach in toward the spine, up to the left rib cage, and then to the left lung. Push your left shoulder and side slightly towards the front.

(2) Inhale a sip of air, pull up the left anus toward the left lung as you pull up the sexual organs. Pull up the left kidney, and then pull up the spleen. Feel the left kidney and the spleen assisting the left lung. Contract the muscles around the left lung, and draw the Chi up to and around that lung through the lower organs.

(3) Pull the Chi up from the left side of the anus to the bladder, left kidney, adrenal gland and spleen until you feel the lung contracting. Feel all of these organs in a line between the lung and the genitals. Use the organs to pull up towards the tongue. Push your tongue hard against the roof of your mouth as you draw the Chi up through the organs to the left lung.

Use the same procedure with the right side until the same line can be felt passing through the associated organs, such as the liver, to your right lung. When you feel the fascial connection to the genitals, use all of the lower organs to pull the genitals up toward the lungs, helping them lift the weights. Once you can exert this power from the lungs, you may eliminate the procedure of expanding the stomach area. (Figure 5-28)

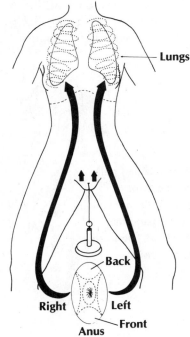

FIGURE 5-28
Inhale and pull up the right and left sides of the anus, directing the energy to the lungs. Wrap the energy around the lungs

NOTE: Don't use force. Use your Chi to lift the weight in conjunction with light muscular action and strong mental power.

d. LIFTING WITH THE HEART—CAUTIOUSLY

As you progress to the heart, be sure that you are in control of the other organs first. The heart and lungs can easily become congested with energy, causing chest pain and difficult breathing. If you have this problem, tap the area around the heart and practice the Healing Sound associated with that organ. (The Six Healing Sounds are described in Appendix 1 and in the book, *Taoist Ways to Transform Stress into Vitality.*)

Before lifting the weight, practice drawing up the Chi and wrapping it into and around the heart. Proceed as follows with caution:

(1) Create a ball of energy in the center of the stomach, above the navel. Inhale a sip of air, pull up the front part of the anus, and expand the "Chi Ball" upward towards the rib cage. Inhale another sip, draw the Chi Ball inward, and then pull it up under the sternum. Expand it under the sternum towards the back and to the left side. Push your tongue up against the roof of your mouth, push the left shoulder towards the front, and feel your heart. (Figure 5-29) Slowly exhale, and regulate your breath.

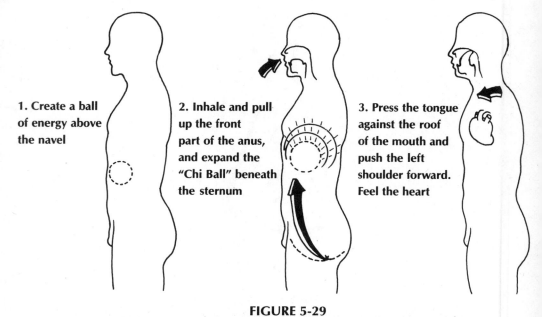

1. Create a ball of energy above the navel

2. Inhale and pull up the front part of the anus, and expand the "Chi Ball" beneath the sternum

3. Press the tongue against the roof of the mouth and push the left shoulder forward. Feel the heart

FIGURE 5-29
The Chi Ball

(2) When you are well practiced, eliminate the step of expanding the stomach area. Simply inhale in sips, pull up the front part of the anus as you pull up the sexual organs. Pull up the stomach to the rib cage, and pull the Chi to the heart, using the power of the heart. Wrap the Chi into and around the heart.

(3) Pull up the genitals, bladder, kidneys, liver, and spleen towards the tongue. Contract the muscles around the heart and lungs, and successively pull the Chi up through each of the lower organs. Start lifting with the lower organs, and draw the Chi upward through each of them to reach the heart.

(4) When you are ready to practice Chi Weight Lifting from the heart, simply pull up the front part of the anus, the genitals, bladder, kidneys, liver, and spleen to the heart. (Figure 5-30) Employ the power of the heart and lungs to help the other organs and glands pull against the genitals, thereby lifting the weight.

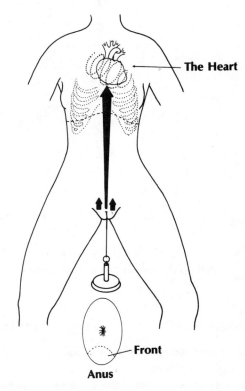

FIGURE 5-30
Pull up the front part of the anus and direct the energy to the heart. Wrap the energy around the heart

e. THE THYMUS GLAND ADDS POWER TO THE HEART AND LUNGS

Sink the sternum to the back as you exhale, and push the lungs towards the thymus under the sternum. Then connect the Chi of the heart to the thymus, which is in close proximity to the heart. Contracting the muscles around the thymus, heart and lungs will greatly increase their combined force, enabling them to draw Chi up through the lower organs, pull up the genitals, and lift the weight. (Figure 5-31)

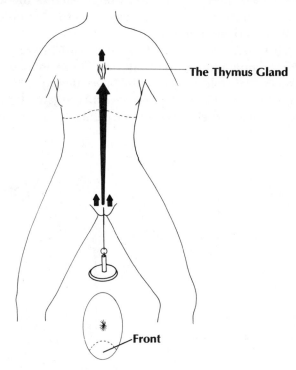

The Thymus Gland

Front

FIGURE 5-31
Pull up the weight by contracting the thymus

f. PULLING FROM THE PITUITARY AND PINEAL GLANDS

The tongue and eyes act as major tools in exerting control over the pituitary and pineal glands.

(1) Practice first by pressing the tongue to the palate, and turn the eyes upward.

(2) Contract the eye muscles towards the middle of the brain to the pituitary gland.

(3) Contract the cranium from all sides: Squeeze in from the crown, the base of the lower jaw near the throat, the front, back, and left and right sides of the skull, gently compressing the center of the brain. Concentrating on the center point behind the "third eye," prepare to draw the energy up to the pituitary gland. (Figure 5-32) You are using the muscles of the skull to increase the pressure on this area.

(4) Contract the middle part of the anus, and pull the Chi all the way up into the brain.

(5) Contract the lungs, heart and thymus gland, and push their energy up towards the center of the brain. The pituitary gland pulls energy from the thymus gland, heart, lungs, spleen, liver, adrenal glands, kidneys, bladder, and sexual organs. All of these parts will then work together to pull up the weight.

(6) Repeat the practice, now focusing on the pineal gland at the crown of the head.

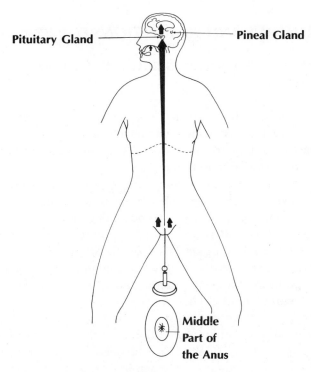

FIGURE 5-32
Contract the middle part of the anus, and pull up all the way to the brain. Lift the weight by contracting the pituitary gland

g. CIRCULATE THE MICROCOSMIC ORBIT

Since all the steps of this exercise are extremely powerful, use caution. The Microcosmic Orbit meditation is a very important safety measure. When finished with all of these steps, circulate the energy in the Microcosmic Orbit several times, collecting it in the navel. Finally, remove the weight.

6. Finish Chi Weight Lifting

After you have released the weights, practice the Power Lock two or three times up to the crown, and massage the sexual organs again. First massage the genitals, sacrum, and perineum with the cloth, then practice the Sexual Energy Massage techniques. As stated earlier, the Healing Tao is not responsible for your use or misuse of this practice. THE MASSAGE TECHNIQUES ARE YOUR BEST PROTECTION. DO NOT NEGLECT THEM AT ANY TIME.

F. PRECAUTIONS AND SUGGESTIONS FOR PRACTICE

NOTE: THE BEST PRECAUTION IS COMMON SENSE. READ THIS SECTION CAREFULLY!

Although most of these suggestions are directed at men because they are at a greater risk, women can also be affected in adverse ways by this practice if they are not careful. Read all of the following precautions to fully understand this practice.

1. Be sure that the Microcosmic Orbit is clear of any blockages.

2. MEN AND WOMEN: Be well versed in all of the prerequisites before attempting this practice. Without a degree of mastery of Iron Shirt Chi Kung I, a student may not be grounded enough to safely accumulate external energies. Without the Six Healing Sounds, the organs may overheat. Without the Microcosmic Orbit Meditation, there is no point in doing any practice taught in this system. Trouble would be the only result.

3. MEN: If you have not mastered the Sexual Power Lock, and therefore cannot prevent an ejaculation, you should not practice Chi Weight Lifting. Practice Healing Love instead. If you have mastered these techniques, but you lose your seminal fluid accidentally, abstain from Chi Weight Lifting for at least two to three days after the accident. Be prepared to drastically reduce the weight you would nor-

mally lift, since Chi diminishes with the loss of seminal fluid, making the practice unsafe. (See Appendix 1.) Further information is available in the book, *Taoist Secrets of Love; Cultivating Male Sexual Energy*.

NOTE: It is safe to practice Chi Weight Lifting after sex, provided that the seminal fluid is retained. You should still be prepared to reduce the weight, however, if the act of sex drains you in any way.

4. WOMEN: If you have not mastered the Orgasmic Draw, do so before you practice Chi Weight Lifting. Although Chi Weight Lifting is actually safer for women than it is for men, less Chi will be available for the internal organs to pull the weight if too much sexual energy is expended. The remedy is not celibacy, but rather the practice of the Orgasmic Draw. (See Appendix 1.) Further information can be found in the book, *Healing Love Through the Tao: Cultivating Female Sexual Energy*.

5. Women should NEVER continue Chi Weight Lifting during a menstrual period, vaginal infection, or at any stage of pregnancy. When these times have passed, practice may be resumed. Wait at least two or three days until after menstruation has finished.

6. MEN AND WOMEN: The ancient Taoist masters advised that one abstain from sex for the first one hundred days of this practice. For the best results in the modern world, abstain at least until you have comfortably mastered the lightest weights. DO NOT TRY TO SPEED UP YOUR PROGRESS FOR THIS PURPOSE. This is recommended because men and women must fully retain their sexual energy before they can safely practice Chi Weight Lifting.

7. MEN AND WOMEN: Take extra care not to allow the accumulation of too much sexual energy in the head. Headaches, numbness, or discomfort can be alleviated by pressing the tongue to the roof of the mouth and drawing the pressure out of the head, down through the tongue, and into the navel. Spiral the energy, following the same procedures used at the end of the Microcosmic Orbit Meditation.

8. Remember that the Genital Compression exercises found in Chapter Three are the best ways to replenish the sexual energy you are extracting from the ovaries or testicles. Use this after the Chi Weight Lifting practice.

9. Men may find, upon mastering Chi Weight Lifting, their Power Draw is so powerful that the testicles are drawn into the body after the weights are removed. DO NOT BE ALARMED. No harm will come of this, provided that you relax and don't cause yourself any harm

through fear or rash action. You may employ the Genital Compression technique, but it is not absolutely necessary. The testicles descend by themselves within a few minutes or, at the most, a few hours.

In ancient times it was considered a priceless asset for a male martial artist to be able to retract his testicles into the body to avoid having them crushed or damaged by an opponent. In spiritual circles, this was a valued practice because the maintenance of Ching Chi could no longer tax the organs and glands if no sperm were produced. (The testicles cannot produce sperm in a retracted state.) Taoist adepts who practice to this end will eventually acquire full access to their internal energy.

NOTE FOR MEN AND WOMEN: Sexual energy transforms into life-force energy, which transforms into spiritual energy. The ability to stop the actual production of sperm or eggs means there is one less transformation for energy to go through, since life-force energy becomes directly available. This should not be taken to mean that such a practice is being advocated, but to inform you of its ramifications. The ancient masters saw this as a short-cut to the cultivation of spiritual energy, leaving one with fewer steps to cover on the spiritual path.

10. MEN: Never try to lift weights without using the entire groin. The cloth must be tied around the penis and the testicles together. Using the testicles alone defies common sense; however, there are those who can be tempted to try new things without first reading the instructions.

11. MEN: Never lift weights with an erection. This can lead to a great deal of pain as the pressure of the weight expands into the already engorged head of the penis. Further, lifting with an erection may create conditions which can lead to blood clots.

12. MEN: To help prevent painful slippage of the cloth, tighten the knot at the base of the testicles so that it almost touches the perineum. Try to avoid too much slack around the groin while lifting, but do not cut off circulation.

13. In the beginning stages of practice, a man might feel a little pain in the groin or in the abdomen caused by the lifting of the weight. Massage very carefully before and after Chi Weight Lifting, and follow the procedures with caution. The massage should reduce any pain you may experience.

NOTE: Once your sexual organs become stronger, the pain gradually goes away. This is not unlike the muscle pain that occurs in normal weight lifting. Some may experience fever; however, there have been no reports of infections of the testes resulting from this practice. You may wish to use only the massage techniques until the pain stops, and then resume lifting.

14. MEN AND WOMEN: If you feel pain in your internal organs after training, practice the Microcosmic Orbit Meditation and the Six Healing Sounds until the pain is gone. The pain may be a sign of overheating which means that Chi Weight Lifting should be discontinued until the pain subsides. This may also be an indication that your internal organs are not in a healthy condition. If so, resume practicing the less advanced techniques instead of Chi Weight Lifting until you can comfortably lift weights.

15. **WARNING FOR MEN:** If you know that you already have a blood clot from circumstances which pre-date this practice, consult a physician about the severity of the problem before attempting Chi Weight Lifting.

A blood clot should be fully dissipated for complete safety in these practices. Otherwise, it can dislodge and relocate in a vital area bringing serious or lethal consequences. A medical consultation should reveal whether or not the Sexual Energy Massage or Chi Weight Lifting techniques can be safely used with an existing blood clot. If not, ask your doctor about options to help circumvent or alleviate the problem. There are medical methods of eliminating blood clots. The Healing Tao is not responsible for your choice, however. Your physician's advice and your internal sensitivities must be your guidelines in such matters.

16. MEN AND WOMEN: If you scratch the skin of the sexual organs, clean the area, and allow it to heal before you do this practice. You can practice Hitting with the massage techniques, but it is best to avoid lifting weights if the groin is hurt. You may apply medications that you have used before, providing that the sexual organs are kept dry. (Hydrogen peroxide is useful for keeping a wound clean and dry.) Men should avoid using most medications on or around the sensitive tip of the penis.

17. WOMEN: See a physician or gynecologist for wounds within the vaginal wall that require medication. Do not use any medications internally without a doctor's advice.

18. Although it is better to lift less weight for longer periods of time

than to lift heavier weights for shorter periods, avoid lifting any weight for more than 60 seconds. Men in particular must avoid cutting off the circulation of blood to the testicles.

19. Do not try to outdo yourself or anyone else because you then stand a good chance of getting hurt. If you feel any strain at all, REMOVE THE WEIGHTS IMMEDIATELY.

20. If you haven't practiced for more than a week, do not return to the same weight you were able to lift before the layoff. Build up again slowly to avoid injuring yourself.

NOTE: When energy is low, and you still choose to practice, spend more time massaging the genitals, and less time hanging the weight. (Women should massage the breasts as well.) When you have finished Chi Weight Lifting, hit your hands, legs and back only. For at least two or three days refrain from striking areas where the impact might reach vital organs, or wait until you again feel alert and vigorous.

21. When some people detoxify, diarrhea, nausea, or pain in some of the organs may result as they are cleansed by the process. These are all temporary; however, Chi Weight Lifting and Hitting can also initiate some long term effects which are ultimately good:

a. During the first 100 days of practice, a reduced sex drive may result from the sexual energy transferring up to the higher centers to heal the organs and glands. Once the body has had a chance to repair itself, the sexual energy will increase greatly, thereby restoring the sex drive.

b. A need to drink more water may result from changes in one's metabolism.

c. Practice may cause either an increase or loss of appetite, accompanied by exhaustion. This may be part of the re-balancing process that the body goes through as energy is being assimilated. Some overweight people begin to lose weight; some underweight people find that they are eating more.

d. When you practice Chi Weight Lifting you may feel heat, muscle spasms, shakiness, coldness, breezes, or simply an overall "funny" feeling. The body may not yet be adjusted to the increase in Chi, or the energy may be fighting diseases in the body, thereby causing such symptoms. Use your own judgment as to whether you should continue the process, but if serious physical problems persist, consult your doctor.

e. As certain levels of practice are attained, some people dream profusely. This may be because they are practicing Chi Weight Lifting and Hitting in excess, or they may be Hitting too hard. This causes the organs to overheat. Also, if the physical body is too hard and tight, emotions may be locked in the muscles and organs. The Hitting process may release them. Pain felt in the tendons and muscles can cause a great deal of dreaming. The increase in Chi, and its fight against diseases of the body, can cause great internal changes which may also be the source of excessive dreaming.

22. Be especially careful if you suffer from high blood pressure. The Power Draw and Orgasmic Draw can raise the blood pressure considerably if you do not have your Microcosmic Orbit opened sufficiently. If the Microcosmic Orbit is open and flowing, the blood pressure can be reduced and eventually controlled.

23. Do not practice Chi Weight Lifting and Hitting on a full stomach. Wait at least one hour after a meal before practicing. Also, to keep from losing Chi when you have finished exercising, do not eat for one-half hour to an hour.

24. Do not shower right away after practice, especially if you sweat. Allow your body to cool down for a while. You are still absorbing Chi at this point; therefore, it is better to avoid washing away external energy.

25. MEN: If you have washed before practicing, be sure to dry yourself thoroughly. Otherwise, you may abrade yourself if your skin is still moist when you apply the weight.

26. MEN: You may wish to cut your pubic hair short. If it is left long, pain may result since it is pulled during Chi Weight Lifting.

27. Urinate or have a bowel movement before practice. If this is not possible, try to wait one or two hours after practice before fulfilling these functions in order to prevent any loss of accumulated Chi. This will give the body time to absorb the Chi into the bones, organs, and glands. Collect the energy in the navel.

28. In hot weather, do not drink too much cold water because the body must expend a great deal of internal energy to warm it. This may result in too much cold energy in the heart, which can be harmful.

29. Many people have reported a loss of desire for alcohol, drugs, tobacco, coffee, and tea as a result of the detoxification initiated by Chi Weight Lifting and Hitting. It is best to avoid these toxic substances in any case, but keep in mind that they will satisfy you less if you detoxify faster than these substances are taken in. The stimulation they offer may not occur if they are forced out of the body before they can affect you.

30. Do not stand on a cold floor during practice. If there is no rug,

stand on a towel. A cold floor will draw away your energy.

31. In the early stages, avoid practicing at night, because you may not be able to sleep. When you become proficient, you should be able to practice at any time.

32. Remember that the purpose of your training is to raise your energy levels and to rid your body of toxins. It is NOT to promote violence or foolishness. Do not walk into your local bar and make claims to being the sexual weight lifting champion of the Healing Tao. You may find that this particular subject is not well received in certain social atmospheres.

33. Be aware that practices that draw sexual energy into the body can spread any existing venereal infection. Be sure that you are free of such problems before attempting the Sexual Energy Massage or Chi Weight Lifting.

34. **WARNING FOR MEN AND WOMEN:** Be aware of your body's reactions to Chi Weight Lifting. Although this system is known for its many safeguards to avoid side effects, it is difficult to account for the internal differences in people. ANY problems that do not appear to be covered in this book must be directed to the Healing Tao. In such cases, Chi Weight Lifting should be discontinued until you are fully aware of your status.

G. SUMMARY OF CHI WEIGHT LIFTING

1. Pre-Chi Weight Lifting Exercises:
   a. Increasing Chi Pressure: Practice from nine to 81 times.
   b. Increasing Kidney Pressure: Practice from six to 36 times.
   c. Power Lock Exercise: Practice two to three times up to the crown.
   d. Cloth Massage of Sexual Center, Perineum, and Sacrum
   e. Sexual Energy Massage:

MEN:
   (1) Finger Massage of the Testicles
   (2) Palm Massage of the Testicles
   (3) Ducts Elongation Rubbing
   (4) Stretching the Ducts Gently with Massage
   (5) Stretching the Scrotum and Penis Tendons
   (6) Tapping the Testicles

WOMEN:
    (1) Breast Massage
    (2) Massage the Glands with Accumulated Chi
    (3) Massage the Organs with Accumulated Chi
    (4) Massage the Ovaries
    (5) Internal Egg Exercise (optional)

2. Chi Weight Lifting

a. Prepare the weight on the floor or a chair. (Women: After inserting the string through the egg, tie it to the weight or the weight apparatus.)

b. MEN: Fold the cloth, and tie it around the penis and testicles. Then tie one end of the cloth to the weight holding apparatus.

c. WOMEN: Insert the egg into the vagina, larger end first.

NOTE FOR MEN AND WOMEN: Always hold the weight or the cloth with your hands while standing up to assume a weight lifting posture. Test the weight with the index and middle fingers before releasing it.

d. While testing the weight with your fingers, pull up the left and right sides of the anus to the left and right kidneys respectively, and contract the perineum.

e. If it does not feel too heavy, gently release the string or cloth from the fingers, and hold the weight with the genitals.

f. Swing the weight from 30 to 60 times, inhaling as you pull up with each forward swing. Exhale as the weight moves backward.

g. First lift the weight from each station of the Microcosmic Orbit. (You will actually be lifting the weight using the power of your mind.)

h. Rest as you hold the weight manually, or place it on a high surface, such as a table top. (You may prefer to remove it while resting, and then attach it again to resume lifting.) Collect the energy in the navel during the rest period.

i. Gently release the weight between your legs once again to lift it with the power of the organs and glands, starting with the kidneys.

j. MEN: Lower the weight to the chair or the floor, and untie the cloth from the holding apparatus. Then remove the cloth from the groin.

k. WOMEN: Lower the weight to the chair or the floor, and then remove the egg.

3. MEN AND WOMEN: Practice the Power Lock exercise two or three times up to the crown.

4. Cloth Massage of the Sexual Center, Perineum, and Sacrum

5. Sexual Energy Massage

NOTE: Men in particular should repeat at least two or three of the aforementioned massage techniques to replenish the circulation of blood in the sexual center, and to help dissipate any coagulation which can lead to blood clots. Women repeat the same procedures at their own pace.

6. Hitting (See Chapter Four.)

7. Use at least two or three of the Six Healing Sounds, especially the Heart and Lung Sounds. All of them are useful if you have the time to do them.

8. Practice the Microcosmic Orbit meditation for several minutes. In conjunction with this meditation, you can also practice Bone Breathing. Use your mind to absorb the released Ching Chi into the bones.

Chapter Six

SUMMARY

This chapter is both a summary of Bone Marrow Nei Kung and a sample of its use with other Taoist physical disciplines. You may tailor your own training schedule from this information provided that you have thoroughly studied each exercise, and you know the precautions associated with each. DO NOT START TRAINING UNTIL YOU HAVE FULLY UNDERSTOOD THE PREVIOUS CHAPTERS.

When practiced together, these exercises can be completed within 45 minutes in an abbreviated format. There are nine distinct disciplines in this particular schedule. The Inner Smile, Microcosmic Orbit, Healing Love, Iron Shirt Chi Kung I, and the Six Healing Sounds are included as part of the regimen. When some degree of proficiency has been reached, practice according to your needs; however, do not neglect any of these disciplines entirely.

A. THE BEGINNER'S APPROACH TO BONE MARROW NEI KUNG

In the beginning, people are apprehensive about the time and effort required to achieve goals within this system. Indeed, the regimen may appear overwhelming to a novice. Similar questions arise among experienced practitioners, but for a different reason. The concern of the novice is how to create the time for such an esoteric discipline. The concern of the adept is that nothing interfere with the time allotted for practice.

Obviously, the most difficult task is getting started. People spend twelve to eighteen years obtaining the education they need to create the best possible foundation for a career, family, and social life. In the process they must often temporarily neglect their physical and spiritual health in favor of earning a living. The need for entertainment and social interaction often compounds the situation. Eventually, you must consider just how "temporary" the situation really is concerning your health and well-being.

Once Bone Marrow Nei Kung is established as a daily regimen, people often find more time, energy, and pleasure in their lives. Internal health provides a wider range of capabilities and increased efficiency in your daily functions. The cultivation of internal power leads first to self-healing, then to radiant health, and ultimately to a better overall perspective. In this system, you will learn how to improve your capabilities to create more time for the pleasures of life.

B. THE GENERAL FEATURES OF TRAINING

1. The Inner Smile is the most important aspect of early Taoist training because it draws positive energy to the internal organs and glands. It is taught as part of the Microcosmic Orbit meditation, but it is also distinct in that the Inner Smile makes new energy accessible through the mid eyebrow and the eyes. The Microcosmic Orbit is actually the pathway through which the associated meditation circulates internally stored energy while distributing new energy absorbed from the Inner Smile.

2. The Microcosmic Orbit Meditation should be used as part of the Bone Marrow Nei Kung regimen as well as being practiced regularly by itself. In this meditation energy is circulated through twelve stations located along two major pathways of the body. The first extends from the palate to the perineum, and the second extends from the perineum to the crown, returning to the palate through the mid-eyebrow. With the Inner Smile, this meditation should be practiced in the morning before your day begins and, along with the Six Healing Sounds, in the evening to decelerate the body.

3. The Healing Love is crucial to Bone Marrow Nei Kung in order to prevent the loss of sexual energy. The practice includes a sexual version of the Power Lock, the Genital Compression exercise, and Testicle/Ovarian Breathing. (The Sexual Power Lock is explained in Appendix 1.) In Bone Marrow Nei Kung, the Power Lock is used without any sexual arousal to draw Ching Chi into the Microcosmic Orbit. The Sexual Power Lock prevents the loss of Ching Chi during sex by drawing this energy into the body rather than expelling it. This also reduces the energy loss suffered by women during menstruation.

4. Iron Shirt I can be simplified to accommodate some of the Bone Marrow Nei Kung exercises, such as Bone Breathing and Bone Com-

pression, which can be initiated from the "Embracing the Tree" posture. Unless you wish to emphasize Iron Shirt Chi Kung I in your regimen, the other five postures can be done later in the day, or whenever you feel more ambitious about your training. It is useful for rooting the body and drawing energy from the earth. Refer to the book, *Iron Shirt Chi Kung I* for the complete practice.

5. Bone Breathing and Bone Compression can be practiced anywhere as separate exercises, or to initiate Bone Marrow Nei Kung. Simply inhale, pack, spiral, and squeeze Chi successively into the limbs and the body from a seated position, or from the "Embracing the Tree" posture of Iron Shirt Chi Kung I. You may also use Bone Breathing and Bone Compression as part of the Hitting practice, combining them for the ultimate compression of sexual and external energy into the body.

6. The Sexual Energy Massage releases Ching Chi from the sexual center into the Microcosmic Orbit to be disseminated throughout the body and compressed into the bones. It is the primary practice because it is extremely powerful when combined with Healing Love techniques, and it is much safer than Chi Weight Lifting. The exercises related to the Sexual Energy Massage techniques are the Power Lock (non-sexual), Genital Compression and the Preliminary Cloth Massage. These prepare the genitals by stimulating the Ching Chi for its ascension into the body. They also replenish the circulation of blood and Chi in the sexual center after practice.

7. As stated throughout this text, Chi Weight Lifting is documented for those students who have received the necessary training. The Sexual Energy Massage techniques will suffice for the purposes of Bone Marrow Nei Kung, and they must certainly be mastered prior to attempting this practice. Chi Weight Lifting differs from the massage techniques in that it further strengthens the fasciae which connect the genitals to the internal organs and glands. This is achieved by lifting light weights, and gradually increasing the length of time they are held, but never exceeding sixty seconds.

NOTE: Do not neglect the Power Lock, Cloth Massage, and Sexual Energy Massage techniques before and after Chi Weight Lifting.

8. The Hitting practice has two forms: one uses a wire device, the other uses rattan sticks. (Either can be used with packing.) The first form initiates strong vibrations, opening the pores of the bones to absorb new energies while detoxifying the system. The second form strengthens the nervous system by increasing the skin's tolerance for

external contact while stimulating lymphocyte production used in the creation of antibodies.

9. The Six Healing Sounds should complete the training in order to release trapped tension and excess heat from the body. These sounds are practiced from a seated posture after the Hitting techniques and the Microcosmic Orbit meditation. They serve to decelerate the body since its metabolic rate will be extremely high by the end of a Bone Marrow Nei Kung training session.

NOTE: The Microcosmic Orbit meditation still takes precedence over all other facets of this regimen. If you have little time for meditation, spend less time on each discipline; otherwise, do not practice until you can make the time for both the practice and the meditation.

C. A SAMPLE TRAINING SCHEDULE

At this point you have enough information on each practice to combine them into a Bone Marrow Nei Kung regimen. This summary is intended to help you assimilate what you have learned into your practice. Keep the book nearby and open to this page when you are ready to begin.

1. The Inner Smile

a. Sit on the edge of a chair with your hands held together and eyes closed.

b. Re-create a happy emotional state, and express it with your best smile. Also smile by lifting the outer corners of your eyelids to enhance the process.

c. Picture a radiant smile of energy on the face of a glowing sun directly in front of you.

d. Sense a coolness in your eyes to attract and absorb the warm energy.

e. Mentally enhance the radiance and any color, or perceptions of warmth, until your eyes are filled with it.

f. Let the smiling energy spread down to the organs as you smile to your heart, lungs, liver, spleen, and kidneys. It is your smile that will give the energy its positive charge.

g. Draw in more energy through the mid-eyebrow and the eyes to stimulate the entire system. The process can take up to fifteen minutes before you are ready to circulate the energy in the Microcosmic Orbit.

2. The Microcosmic Orbit (Figure 6-1)

    a. After smiling down, collect the energy at the navel.

    b. Let the energy flow down to the sexual center.

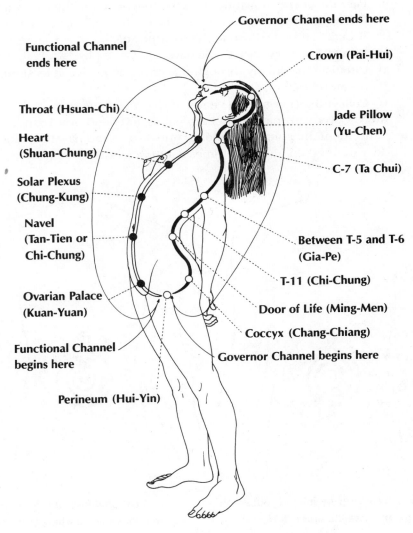

FIGURE 6-1
The Functional and Governor Channels of the Microcosmic Orbit

    c. Move the energy from the sexual center to the perineum.

    d. Draw the energy up from the perineum to the sacrum.

    e. Draw the energy up to the Ming Men, opposite the navel.

    f. Draw the energy up to the T-11 vertebrae.

    g. Draw the energy up to the base of the skull.

    h. Draw the energy up to the crown and circulate it.

    i. Move the energy down from the crown to the mid-eyebrow.

    j. Pass the energy down through the tongue to the throat center.

    k. Bring the energy down from the throat to the heart center.

    l. Bring the energy down to the solar plexus.

    m. Bring the energy back to the navel.

    n. Circulate the energy through this entire sequence at least nine or ten times.

    o. Collect the energy at the navel.

MEN: Cover your navel with both palms, left hand over right. Collect and mentally spiral the energy outward at the navel 36 times clockwise, and then inward 24 times counterclockwise. (Figure 6-2)

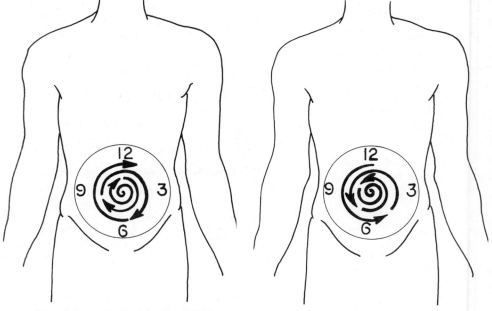

1. Collect the energy by spiraling outwardly from the navel 36 times clockwise

2. Then spiral inwardly 24 times counterclockwise, finishing at the navel

FIGURE 6-2
MEN

WOMEN: Cover your navel with both palms, right hand over left. Collect and mentally spiral the energy outward from the navel 36 times counterclockwise, and then inward 24 times clockwise. (Figure 6-3)

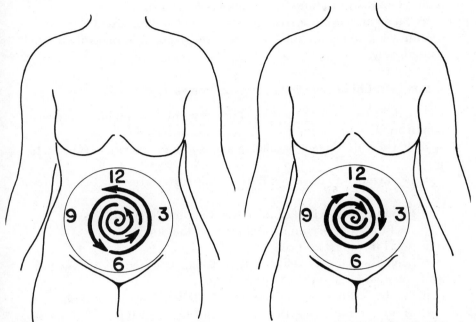

1. Collect the energy by spiraling outwardly from the navel 36 times counterclockwise

2. Then spiral inwardly 24 times clockwise, finishing at the navel

FIGURE 6-3
WOMEN

3. Testicle and Ovarian Breathing

a. Inhale and use mental power and a slight muscular contraction to draw the testicles upward. Hold the energy as you exhale, and slowly lower the testicles. Women inhale, and squeeze the vagina, drawing the energy of the ovaries to the Ovarian Palace.

b. Guide the unaroused sexual energy up through the perineum by inhaling and pulling up the testes or contracting the vagina slightly.

c. Guide the Ching Chi up the back as if sipping on a straw. Slightly arch the lower back outward as if flattening the back against a wall. This will activate the Sacral and Cranial Pumps. Hold the attention at the sacrum and exhale slowly.

d. Relax the sacrum and neck back to their normal positions.

e. Inhale and guide the energy up to T-11 repeating steps 4, 5 and 6.

f. The next stopping place is the Jade Pillow at the base of the skull.

g. Guide the energy up to the head and spiral the energy nine times clockwise and nine times counterclockwise.

h. Men can leave the cold energy in the head for a while. Women should bring the resultant hot energy down the Microcosmic Route immediately.

4. Iron Shirt Chi Kung I: Embracing the Tree Posture

Use this posture for practicing Bone Breathing and Bone Compression, Iron Shirt I techniques, weight lifting, and so on.

a. Stand with the feet parallel at a foot-to-knee distance from each other.

b. Dig firmly into the ground by slightly turning out the balls of the feet.

c. Rotate your pelvis back until the thigh tendons can relax.

d. Feel that the sacrum is pulling the spine down.

e. Relax the chest and ribs.

f. Keep the back as straight as possible. The neck is gently, but firmly pushed back at the C-7 point.

g. Pull back the lower jaw towards the Jade Pillow of the skull.

h. Hold the hands vertically at shoulder level with the fingers spread and the elbows dropped beneath them. Point the fingers towards those of the opposite hand.

i. Position the arms as if they were encircling a tree. Hold the thumbs outward slightly, with the pinkies directed inward, and relax the other fingers.

j. Drop the shoulders, round the scapulae, and sink the chest.

k. Relax the neck, and feel the Chi connecting the hip joints with the knee and ankle joints, and feel their energy connecting with the ground.

5. Bone Breathing and Bone Compression:

NOTE: These may be done in conjunction with Hitting rather than as separate practices.

a. From either a seated position or the posture outlined above, draw in external energy through the fingers as you inhale; release it as you exhale.

b. Inhale and exhale through the lower and upper arms successively. Begin to spiral the energy as you draw it in.

c. Breathe into the toes in the same manner.

d. Continue to breathe into the legs, the pelvis, and spiral the energy.

e. Combine the draw of external energy from both sources and allow them to meet at the spine.

f. Draw the combined energy up to the head, and spiral it.

g. Breathe the energy into the ribs and sternum from the spine, and continue to spiral it.

h. Inhale, spiral, pack, and squeeze into all sections simultaneously; hold your breath as you compress the energy into your bones; then exhale.

6. The Sexual Energy Massage

a. THE POWER LOCK

The Power Lock is practiced before and after the Sexual Energy Massage to assist in the upward draw of the released energy and sexual hormones. It employs nine short sips of breath with nine contractions of the genital, anal and perineal areas. The tongue is pushed against the palate, and the buttocks and teeth are clenched to activate the Cranial and Sacral Pumps. Together with these contractions, the three middle fingers of either hand are used to press a point at the back of the perineum, near the anus, to help guide the rising energy up to the five stations of the sacrum, T-11 point, C-7 point, base of the skull, and the crown point. The goal is to draw sexual energy from the perineum to the crown.

b. GENITAL COMPRESSION

This exercise replenishes the energy drawn from the genitals during the other practices. This is not a Bone Marrow Nei Kung technique in itself, but rather a separate practice for use afterwards. The method compresses energy into the genitals of men or women to increase their production of Ching Chi.

c. THE PRELIMINARY CLOTH MASSAGE

A silk cloth is used to massage in circular motions the genital area, perineum, coccyx, and sacrum. This is used before and after the Sexual Energy Massage to first prepare the genitals for the exercise, and then later to replenish the flow of blood and Chi to the sexual center. This is particularly useful in preventing blood coagulation and subsequent blood clots from occurring in the genitals of male practitioners.

d. THE SEXUAL ENERGY MASSAGE FOR MEN

    (1) Finger Massage of the Testicles
    (2) Palm Massage of the Testicles
    (3) Ducts Elongation Rubbing
    (4) Stretching the Ducts Gently with Massage
    (5) Stretching the Scrotum and Penis Tendons
    (6) Tapping the Testicles

e. THE SEXUAL ENERGY MASSAGE FOR WOMEN

    (1) Breast Massage
    (2) Massage of the Glands with Accumulated Chi
    (3) Massage of the Organs with Accumulated Chi
    (4) Massage the Ovaries

f. THE INTERNAL EGG EXERCISE

This exercise uses a jade egg to resist internal contractions of the vaginal canal, thereby strengthening its three sections. The first section is the front of the vaginal canal, within the external orifice. The second section is the middle of the canal between the first and third sections. The third section is directly beneath the cervix, near the end of the canal.

7. Chi Weight Lifting for Men and Women

As you swing the weights, first pull them from the Microcosmic Orbit as the energy flow resisting the pressure of the weights passes through the perineum, sacrum, T-11 and C-7 vertebrae, Jade Pillow, and crown. Later, as you continue to lift from the perineum, both sides of the anus should be pulled up as you pack Chi around both kidneys. Starting at the kidneys, lift from the lower organs successively upwards, eventually employing the higher organs, and finally lift from the pineal and pituitary glands. Circulate the released energy through the Microcosmic Orbit upon removing the weights.

a. Start with the Power Lock, Cloth Massage, and Sexual Energy Massage. The weight should be placed on a chair or the floor.

b. Men: Tie the cloth around the entire groin (not the testicles alone). Attach a light weight to the cloth. Women: Attach a light weight to the string held by the egg, then insert the egg into the vagina.

c. Lift the weight from its resting place, and swing it, using the strength of the Microcosmic Orbit to create the upward force. Begin by pulling up the front, middle, and back anus to bring the Chi to the sacrum from where it will be pulled up the spine to the head. Use every station of the Microcosmic Orbit to assist in pulling the weight.

d. Concentrate on the kidneys. Pull up the right and left anus as you wrap Chi around the kidneys, and then lift the weight from the kidneys.

e. Pull up the right and left anus. Wrap Chi around the spleen and the liver. Pull the weight from the spleen and the liver.

f. Use the same procedure to lift from the lungs. Pull the weights from a straight line through the organs beneath each lung.

g. Pull up as you contract the heart, lungs, spleen, liver, adrenals, kidneys, and thereby the weights. Feel the fascial connection between all of these organs and the genitals.

h. Add the strength of the thymus gland to the upward draw of the organs.

i. Finally, press the tongue to the palate, pull up both sides of the anus, contract the muscles of the skull, and lift from the pituitary and pineal glands through all of the previous organs.

j. After you release the weights, repeat the Power Lock exercise, Cloth Massage, and Sexual Energy Massage.

8. Hitting with Packing

Inhale, spiral, pack, and squeeze external and sexual energy into each area as you prepare to apply the Hitting device; hold the breath and muscle tension as you hit; then exhale and release the tension. When Hitting with the rattans, avoid contact with the spine.

a. Preliminary Hitting: To stimulate energies and detoxify, hit three times the lower Tan Tien (below the navel), the Ming Men (opposite the navel on the spine), the inside of both elbows, and the backs of both knees. This is optional when using the rattans.

b. Hit the five abdominal lines.

c. Hit the rib cage and the sternum very lightly at an angle.

d. Hit the three lines of the back (two lines with the rattans).

e. Hit the left and right sides of the body.

f. Gently tap the head and jaw.

g. Hit the four lines of each arm: the Middle Finger Line, the Thumb Line, the Back of the Hand Line, and the Pinky Line.

h. Hit the four lines of the legs: The Middle Line (down the front), the Big Toe Line, the Small Toe Line, and the Back of the Leg Line.

9. The Six Healing Sounds

Do the Lung Sound and the Heart Sound as described in Appendix 1. The other four sounds and related postures are optional, but they are useful in helping the body to decelerate at the end of this regimen. You may wish to begin any of the higher level meditations, or else practice the Inner Smile and Microcosmic Orbit again.

10. Combining the Practices

When you are well acquainted with the supplemental disciplines, you can combine them into one practice from the Embracing the Tree posture.

a. Assume the Embracing the Tree posture.

b. Smile down to the organs, glands, and navel.

c. Practice "Energizer Breathing" by pushing and pulling the lower abdomen out and in to emphasize each inhalation and exhalation for nine, eighteen, or 36 breaths.

d. Do the three stages of packing for Iron Shirt Chi Kung I as described in Appendix 1.

e. Practice Bone Breathing.

f. Practice Testicle/Ovarian Breathing.

g. Do the Genital Compression exercise two or three times.

h. Do from three to six sets of the Power Lock exercise.

i. Practice the Microcosmic Orbit for three to six rounds.

j. Collect the energy in the navel.

D. PLANNING YOUR PRACTICE

1. Bone Marrow Nei Kung Regimen

a. Ideally, you should begin by spending from fifteen to 30 minutes on the Microcosmic Orbit with the Inner Smile, and ten minutes practicing Iron Shirt Chi Kung I.

b. Begin the Cloth Massage and practice the Power Lock exercise to start the flow of sexual energy to the higher energy centers.

c. Begin the Sexual Energy Massage. Then, providing that you have received training, you may follow the massage techniques with Chi Weight Lifting.

d. Repeat the Power Lock exercise for at least two or three rounds, then repeat the Cloth Massage.

e. Repeat two or three of the Sexual Energy Massage techniques after Chi Weight Lifting to replenish the circulation of blood and Chi in the sexual center, thereby avoiding blood clots in the male genitals.

f. Begin the Hitting practice. Use the bundled wires to create the vibrations that will force the sexual energy into the bones, organs, and glands as you pack and spiral the energy. Rest after you hit each line.

g. Use the rattan sticks to strengthen the skin, muscles, nervous and lymphatic systems. Rest after you hit each line.

h. Finish the entire process with the Microcosmic Orbit Meditation and the Six Healing Sounds.

2. Time for Practice

The best time to practice, as previously mentioned, is in the morning after you have eliminated body wastes and bathed, but you can also practice in the afternoon. You are advised not to practice in the evening because you are creating a great deal of energy, and you may have difficulty sleeping. Try to maintain a specific schedule until you are proficient.

3. Frequency of Practice

In the very beginning practice two to three times a week. Once you are proficient, you may begin to practice on a daily basis. As in all the other Healing Tao disciplines, Chi Weight Lifting and Hitting take time to learn. Eventually, all the steps will begin to blend together into an easily practiced sequence which will increase your energy as your body becomes stronger and healthier.

4. Practice during Travel

The Sexual Energy Massage, Healing Love, Bone Breathing and Bone Compression can be practiced easily while traveling. You can also practice Chi Weight Lifting and Hitting, though it may be hard to carry the weights and devices. The Healing Tao suggests the following to help you maintain these disciplines:

a. The bean bag and rattan sticks are light and should present no problems for travel. If necessary, you may use your hands to hit the

Door of Life point on the back, and the lower Tan Tien point below the navel. Then use the palms to hit the limbs and the body.

b. For Chi Weight Lifting, carry the cloth—or the egg—and a small, strong bag in which you can place an object to serve as a weight. Always weigh this object on a scale to determine whether or not it is within your capacity to lift.

APPENDIX 1:
SUPPLEMENTAL EXERCISES

Once the Microcosmic Orbit has been opened, a novice can practice Bone Marrow Nei Kung. However, the most benefit is derived from combining this discipline with other aspects of the system. The following is an abridged review only. Each supplemental exercise requires time to master, and each is further described in other Healing Tao books.

NOTE: These disciplines are not presented as part of a regimen or in any specific order for practice.

A. HEALING LOVE

The effects of Bone Marrow Nei Kung are dependent upon the practice of Healing Love, which rechannels sexual energy to heal the internal system. For the purposes of this book, the sexual version of the Power Lock is given because it encompasses the "Power Draw" technique used by men and the "Orgasmic Draw" technique used by women in the Healing Love practice. These exercises are combined with the three finger technique and the internal contractions of the Power Lock to draw Ching Chi into the Microcosmic Orbit.

1. The Power Draw

For men, the practice of orgasmic redirection employs a form of non-ejaculatory sex which results in the highest internal stimulation that can be achieved. The energy that is normally lost during an ejaculation is instead channelled into the body. When it reaches the organs and glands, this energy causes body orgasms that last longer, feel superior, and lack the exhaustion normally felt after sex. The loss of sexual energy through ejaculation deprives the bone marrow of nourishment and depletes the internal organs and glands of one third of their energy. Ejaculation drains energy from the internal system to replace Ching Chi lost with the seminal fluid.

221

2. The Orgasmic Draw

Women who practice the Orgasmic Draw also experience superior orgasms, shorter menstrual periods, and an increase in life-force energy as Ching Chi is retained for use by the body. The problem women face is the loss of enormous quantities of sexual energy through their menstrual periods. This loss can be limited or completely prevented through the Healing Love practice. Further, the exchange of energies during sex becomes far more valuable to a woman when the Yang Chi imparted by her lover is absorbed into her Microcosmic Orbit. Otherwise, the energy received, as well as her own, will be expelled at the end of her cycle and wasted.

3. Health and Sexual Benefits

Not only do the organs retain their full capacity when Ching Chi is saved, but internal energy compounds itself when it is allowed to accumulate on a regular basis. In other words, men and women who consciously save the internal power normally lost during sex will receive a one-third increase in their life-force energy, which accrues regularly with practice. Consider this to be the interest you collect on your savings which is paid off in strength, health, and superior orgasms. The body improves itself regularly through intelligent sex, and the excess energy can be used to fortify every aspect of your life.

4. The Sexual Power Lock Practice

Review the Power Lock exercise of Chapter Three for the proper sequence of contractions. Healing Love is practiced in an aroused state with or without a partner. In solo practice, use several sets of nine short inhalations—"sips"—with nine simultaneous contractions to each station. Continue to repeat this process, drawing the energy up towards the crown. Remember to push the flat part of the tongue against the roof of the mouth as you force the tip of the tongue against the lower jaw behind the teeth. This opens the crown and increases the force of the energy travelling up the spine.

MEN: During the act of sex, reach behind the buttocks to use the three fingertips on the point in front of the anus. (Figure App. 1-1) Apply pressure after each sip of air. In solo practice, use sets of nine contractions until your erection subsides through your drawing power. Repeat this procedure several times. In both cases, maintain the finger pressure if you are near an ejaculation. Do not release it until the urge to expel the semen is gone. Timing is important. If you

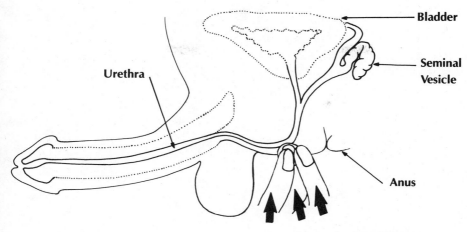

Bladder

Urethra

Seminal
Vesicle

Anus

**Press the urethral opening
in front of the anus**

FIGURE APP. 1-1
**The Sexual Power Lock for men includes pressing against the urethra from a
point at the back of the perineum, in front of the anus**

feel near ejaculation, do not wait to start a set of nine contractions, and be prepared to hold the finger pressure if necessary.

WOMEN: The three fingertips need not be applied by women during the sexual practices. Their main concern is to draw the energy of each orgasm up through the five stations to the crown point, and then to circulate it. (If your Microcosmic Orbit is open, you can draw the energy directly up to the crown.) Finish by storing the energy in the navel. In solo practice, always begin by drawing Ching Chi from the ovaries and sexual center into the perineum. Do not allow it to remain in the sexual center.

MEN AND WOMEN

a. As you initiate the Sexual Power Lock, draw in towards the sacrum with every sip of air. (Men apply the fingers as you hold each contraction.) Pull up the genitals, anus, and perineum, simultaneously clenching the teeth and buttocks. (Figure App. 1-2)

b. Inhale, and pull up the anus to the sacrum. Tilt the sacrum, pull up further to T-11 at the center of the back, opposite the solar plexus,

223

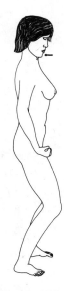

FIGURE APP. 1-2
Initiate the Sexual Power Lock

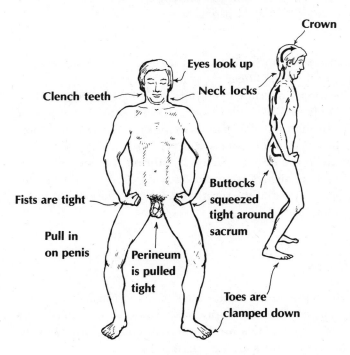

FIGURE APP. 1-3
Inhale and pull all the way up to the crown

and then up to C-7 at the base of the neck. Inhale again, and pull up higher to the base of the skull, and then all the way up to the crown point. (Figure App. 1-3) Spiral the energy, then bring it down to the third eye between the eyebrows, and hold it there for a while.

NOTE: If the Governor channel is completely open, you can draw Ching Chi all the way up to the crown. Always avoid leaving Ching Chi at the Ming Men point opposite the navel because it causes an allergic type of reaction in both kidneys.

    c. Exhale, place the tongue on the palate, and let the energy flow down through the tongue to the throat center. Then bring the energy down to the heart. Rest, and concentrate on the navel. Bring the energy down to the solar plexus, and finally down to the navel. Cover the navel, and spiral the Chi.

    d. Cloth Massage after the Sexual Power Lock: Apply the cloth using circular motions to the perineum, the coccyx, and the sacrum. Starting at the perineum, use the cloth folded lengthwise to massage in a clockwise motion nine to eighteen times, then in a counterclockwise motion nine to eighteen times. Apply the cloth in the same manner to the coccyx, and finally to the sacrum.

NOTE: More information on the Healing Love techniques can be found in the books, *Taoist Secrets of Love: Cultivating Male Sexual Energy* and *Healing Love Through the Tao: Cultivating Female Sexual Energy.*

B. IRON SHIRT CHI KUNG I

1. Energizer Breathing

Begin with Abdominal Breathing (also known as Energizer Breathing) by expanding the lower abdomen on all sides like a ball as you inhale. Breathe into both kidneys and lower the diaphragm as you inhale, making sure to keep the chest relaxed and sunk down. As you exhale, flatten the abdomen completely. Regulate this breathing using quick, short sips to inhale and exhale.

Reverse Abdominal Breathing is practiced in the opposite manner by extending the abdomen as you exhale and retracting it as you inhale. Keep the chest relaxed throughout. Contract the pelvic and urogenital diaphragms, and slightly pull up the Chi Muscle during these exercises.

NOTE: In Iron Shirt I, packing is initiated by contracting the muscles of a given area as you mentally condense the Chi there. Always breathe through the nose in all Healing Tao exercises.

2. Embracing the Tree

This basic rooting posture is similar to the Horse Stance, which is often used in the practice of Chi Weight Lifting. The Embracing the Tree stance is created as follows: Stand with the feet parallel at a heel-to-knee distance from each other. Dig firmly into the ground by slightly turning out the balls of the feet in a gripping motion. Maintain this force throughout the duration of the posture, and do not curl the toes up. The pelvis is rotated back until the thigh tendons can relax. Feel the sacrum pulling the spine down.

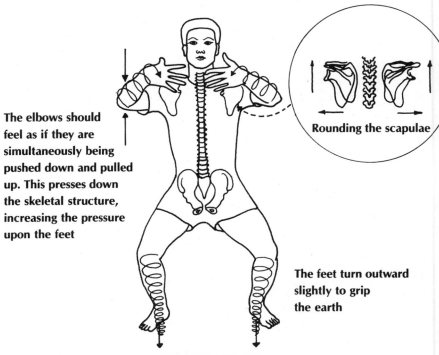

The elbows should feel as if they are simultaneously being pushed down and pulled up. This presses down the skeletal structure, increasing the pressure upon the feet

Rounding the scapulae

The feet turn outward slightly to grip the earth

FIGURE APP. 1-4
Full Embracing the Tree Posture—Front View

Keep the chest relaxed and the back as straight as possible. The neck is gently, but firmly, pushed back at the C-7 point. This is accomplished by pushing back the lower jaw slightly until you feel the C-7 point and the base of the skull aligned with the spine. The head should feel as though it is being lifted from the crown.

The hands are held vertically at shoulder level with the fingers spread and elbows dropped beneath them. Point the fingers towards those of the opposite hand, and position the arms as if they were encircling a tree. Hold the thumbs slightly outward with the pinkies directed inward. Drop the shoulders, joining the scapulae with the spine by rounding the scapulae and sinking the chest. Relax the neck. Feel the connection from the hip joints down to the knee and ankle joints, and feel their connection with the ground. (Figure App. 1-4)

The exercise usually associated with this posture is presented in three stages. If you cannot complete these stages for any reason, it is important that you collect the Chi in the navel. If time does not allow for much work in this area, just use this posture for Bone Breathing and Bone Compression. The actual Iron Shirt I techniques can be done later in a separate practice if necessary.

NOTE: The same precautions for Hitting with Packing apply to this practice. Check with a physician if you have high blood pressure. Women should not use any packing or compression during a menstrual period, or if they are pregnant.

a. STAGE ONE

(1) Assume the posture described above. Press the sacrum down, round the scapulae, relax the chest, and hold the head erect.

(2) Begin Energizer Breathing by pushing and pulling the abdomen out and in to emphasize each inhalation and exhalation. Practice nine to eighteen breaths in this manner.

(3) Exhale, flatten the stomach, and lower the diaphragm. Exhale again, and pull up the pelvic and urogenital diaphragms and the sexual organs.

(4) Inhale in short sips, holding about ten percent of your lung capacity, and tighten the perineum. Sip in twice, and pull up the left and right sides of the anus to the kidneys with each sip. Pack Chi into the kidneys. Do not release the breath until your lungs are comfortably full.

(5) Pull up the sexual organs, sip in air, and pack Chi into the navel. Keep the chest relaxed, and spiral the energy nine times clockwise,

then nine times counterclockwise as you hold the compression around the kidneys and the navel. Do not move your hands.

(6) Breathe into the middle abdomen (one and a half inches below the navel) without spiraling, and pack.

(7) Breathe into the lower abdomen (three inches below the navel) without spiraling, and pack.

(8) Breathe into the perineum, and feel it bulge.

(9) Exhale down through the legs and the feet into the ground approximately six inches. Initiate breathing energy through your palms and soles. Use Energizer Breathing from the lower abdomen for up to eighteen breaths. Feel the energy flowing in the Microcosmic Orbit. (A form of Bone Breathing can also be done at this time.)

b. STAGE TWO

(10) Exhale, flatten the stomach, and pull up the left and right anus. Inhale, tighten the perineum, and squeeze the soles of the feet into the ground. Inhale ten percent of your lung capacity as you pull up the left anus. Hold, and then sip in more air as you pull up the right anus. Pack the kidneys. Claw the toes as though you are gripping the earth, and spiral at the Kidney Points (K-1) on the soles of both feet simultaneously, nine times clockwise and nine times counterclockwise. Use the mind, coordinated with eye movements, to help circulate the energy.

(11) Inhale, bringing the energy from the earth up to the knees. Lock the knees with no spiraling.

(12) Inhale the Chi up to the perineum, and spiral nine times clockwise and nine times counterclockwise. Feel the perineum bulge.

(13) Exhale. Regulate the breath with Energizer Breathing, practice Bone Breathing, and be aware of the soles and palms absorbing and releasing energy. Relax, practice the Inner Smile, and send smiling energy to all of the organs. Feel the energy flow in your Microcosmic Orbit.

c. STAGE THREE

(14) Now exhale again twice and flatten the stomach. Inhale ten percent of your lung capacity, and pull up the front, middle and finally the back part of the anus so that you can direct the Chi into the sacrum. Tilt the sacrum, pack Chi into it, and spiral the energy nine times clockwise and nine times counterclockwise. This will strengthen and activate the Sacral Pump.

(15) Inhale Chi up to T-11, inflating the kidney area, and press out

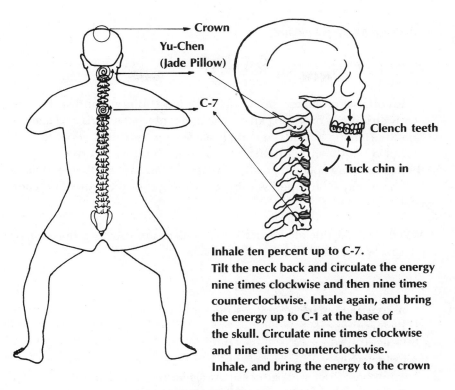

Inhale ten percent up to C-7.
Tilt the neck back and circulate the energy
nine times clockwise and then nine times
counterclockwise. Inhale again, and bring
the energy up to C-1 at the base of
the skull. Circulate nine times clockwise
and nine times counterclockwise.
Inhale, and bring the energy to the crown

FIGURE APP. 1-5
Stage Three of Embracing the Tree

on the lower back to straighten the curve there, spiraling nine times clockwise and nine times counterclockwise.

(16) Inhale up to C-7, straighten the curve at the neck, and lock the neck. Spiral the energy at C-7 nine times clockwise and nine times counterclockwise.

(17) Inhale to the base of the skull. Push the tongue against the palate, clench the teeth tightly, push the chin back, and squeeze the skull and temple bones to activate the Cranial Pump. Spiral nine times clockwise and nine times counterclockwise.

(18) Inhale to the crown (pineal gland) and spiral the energy nine times clockwise and nine times counterclockwise. (Figure App. 1-5)

(19) Concentrate on the space between the eyebrows until you feel Chi build up there. Regulate the breath with Energizer Breathing. Exhale, holding the tongue up to the palate to connect the Governor and Functional channels.

(20) Bring the Chi down through the throat, heart center, and solar plexus. Bring the Chi down to the navel. Collect the energy there by covering the navel with the palms and spiraling in the prescribed manner.

229

C. THE SIX HEALING SOUNDS

Emotional problems, pollution, poor food, injuries, and sudden or overly strenuous exercise can overheat the internal organs and glands. The Six Healing Sounds and their associated postures serve to cool and cleanse the vital organs, stimulating the flow of Chi energy to them. There are specific positions that you can assume to liberate any heat that may be trapped within the cooling sacs that surround each vital organ.

NOTE: Typical side effects of these practices are yawning, burping, or passing wind, all of which are beneficial.

1. Lungs: the First Healing Sound

Associated organ: large intestine
Element: metal
Season: autumn
Color: white
Emotions: Grief and sadness/courage and righteousness
Parts of the body: chest, inner arms, thumbs
Senses: smell (nose) and touch (skin)
Taste: pungent
Sound: SSSSSSSS (tongue behind teeth)
a. Position: Sit up straight on the edge of a chair with the backs of your hands resting on your thighs. (Figure App. 1-6(a)) While looking at your palms, take a deep breath, and raise your arms out in front of you. When the hands are at eye level, begin to rotate the palms and bring them up above your head until the fingers of each hand point toward each other, and the palms face upward and outward. Keep the elbows rounded out to either side. Do not straighten your arms.
b. Sound: Close the jaws so that the teeth meet gently, and part the lips slightly. As you look up, push up through your palms, draw the corners of the mouth back, and exhale the sound "SSSSSSSS" sub-vocally, slowly and evenly in one breath. Picture and feel the sac covering the lungs compress and expel the excess heat, sick energy, sadness, sorrow, and grief. (Figure App. 1-6(b))
c. Rest and Concentrate: When you have exhaled completely, rotate the palms down, gently lowering the shoulders, and slowly lower your hands to your lap, resting them on your thighs, palms up. Close your eyes, and be aware of your lungs, imagining that you are still making the sound. Breathe into the lungs normally to strengthen them. Visu-

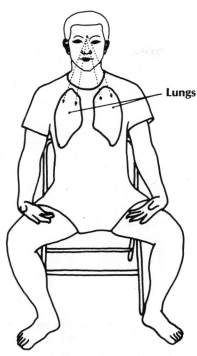

Lungs

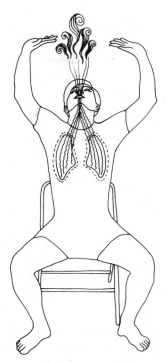

(a) Become aware of the lungs

(b) Picture and feel the sac covering the lungs compress

FIGURE APP. 1-6
The Lungs Sound

alize the color white and smile into the lungs. Try to feel the exchange of cool, fresh energy replacing the hot, wasted energy. Feel righteousness and courage grow within you.

d. Repeat the Lung Sound three to six times. For colds, flu, toothaches, asthma, emphysema, or depression, repeat the exercise six, nine, twelve, or 24 times.

2. Kidneys: the Second Healing Sound

Associated organ: bladder
Element: water
Season: winter
Color: black or dark blue
Emotions: Fear/gentleness
Parts of the body: side of foot, inner legs, chest

231

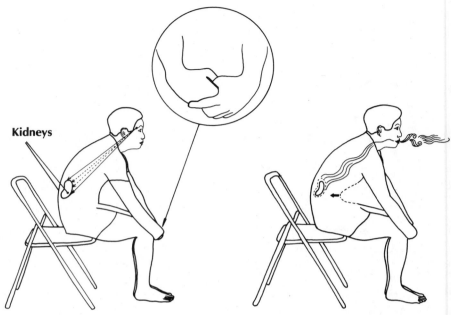

Kidneys

(a) Hook the hands around the knees.
Become aware of the kidneys

(b) Round the lips, making the sound
one makes when blowing out a candle

FIGURE APP. 1-7
The Kidneys Sound

Senses: hearing (ears), bones

Taste: salty

Sound: WOOOOOOO (as when blowing out a candle, the lips forming an "O")

a. Position: Bring your legs together, ankles and knees touching, then take a deep breath and lean forward. Clasp the fingers of your right hand around your left, and embrace your knees with the joined hands. (Figure App. 1-7(a)) Pull back on the arms, straightening them. Allow your back to sag so that it protrudes in the area of your kidneys. Then tilt your head back slightly, and feel the pull on the spine.

b. Sound: Round the lips, and exhale the sound "WOOOOOOO" as if you are blowing out a candle. (Figure App. 1-7(b)) At the same time, contract your abdomen in toward your kidneys. Keep the lips rounded. Imagine the excess heat, the sick energy, and the fear being squeezed out from the membranes surrounding the kidneys.

c. Rest and Concentrate: When you have fully exhaled, sit erect, separate the legs, and place your hands on your thighs with palms up. Close your eyes, breathe into the kidneys, and be aware of them. Visualize the color blue in the kidneys. Smile to them, imagining that you are still making the sound, and feel gentleness there. Be aware of the flowing energy.

d. Repeat the Kidney Sound three to six times. Practice more to alleviate problems of fatigue, dizziness, ringing in the ears, or back pain.

3. Liver: the Third Healing Sound

Associated organ: gall bladder
Element: wood
Season: spring
Color: green
Emotions: anger/kindness
Parts of the body: inner legs, groin, diaphragm, ribs
Senses: sight (eyes), tears
Taste: sour
Sound: SHHHHHHH (tongue near palate)

a. Position: Sit on the edge of your chair, and extend your arms out to the sides, palms up. (Figure App. 1-8(a)) Take a deep breath as you slowly swing your arms up and over your head, following this action with your eyes. Interlace the fingers and turn your joined hands over to face the ceiling, palms up. Push out at the heel of the palms and feel the stretch through the arms into the shoulders. Bend slightly to the left, exerting a gentle pull on the liver.

b. Sound: Open your eyes wide as they are the openings of the liver. Slowly exhale, and sub-vocally emit the sound "SHHHHHHH." Envision the excess heat and anger being expelled from the liver as the sac enveloping the liver is gently compressed. (Figure App. 1-8(b))

c. Rest and Concentrate: When you have fully exhaled, turn the hands over, separate them, and slowly bring the arms down to your sides. Bring the hands to rest on your thighs, palms up. Smile down to the liver. Close your eyes, breathe into the liver, and be aware of it beneath the right rib cage. (Figure App. 1-8(c)) Imagine that you are still making the Liver Sound. Feel kindness grow there and visualize the color green.

d. Repeat the Liver Sound three to six times. Practice more times to expel anger, clear the eyes of any irritations, remove a sour or bitter taste, or to detoxify the liver.

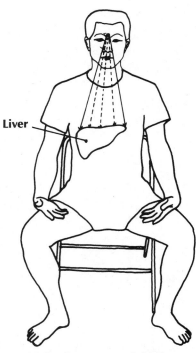

Liver

(a) Become aware of the liver

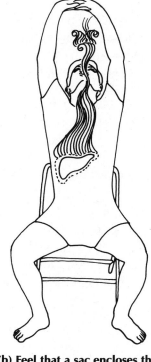
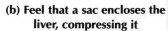

(b) Feel that a sac encloses the liver, compressing it

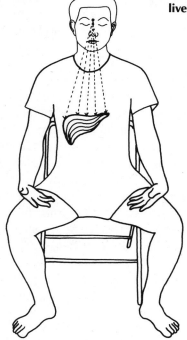

FIGURE APP. 1-8
The Liver Sound

(c) Close your eyes and smile down to the liver

4. Heart: the Fourth Healing Sound

Associated organ: small intestine
Element: fire
Season: summer
Color: red
Emotions: hastiness, arrogance, cruelty/joy, honor, sincerity
Parts of the body: armpits, inner arms
Senses: tongue, speech
Taste: bitter
Sound: HAWWWWWW (mouth wide open)

a. Position: Take a deep breath and assume the same position as for the Liver Sound (Figure App. 1-9(a)), but lean slightly to the right since

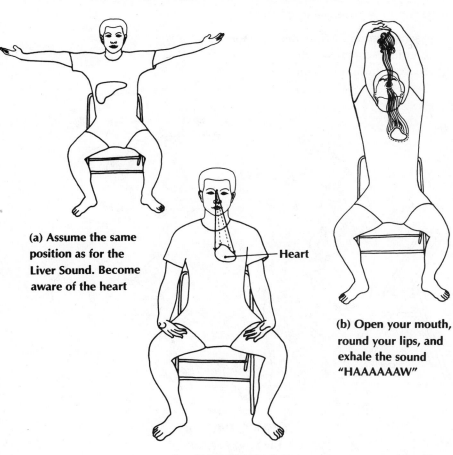

(a) Assume the same position as for the Liver Sound. Become aware of the heart

Heart

(b) Open your mouth, round your lips, and exhale the sound "HAAAAAAW"

FIGURE APP. 1-9
The Heart Sound

235

the heart is located slightly to the left of center in your chest. Focus on the heart and feel the tongue's connection to it.

b. Sound: Open the mouth, round the lips, and exhale the sound "HAWWWWWW" sub-vocally. Picture the sac which surrounds the heart expelling heat, impatience, hastiness, arrogance, and cruelty. (Figure App. 1-9(b))

c. Rest and Concentrate: After exhaling, smile down to the heart, and visualize a bright red color. Feel joy, honor, and sincerity grow in the heart.

d. Repeat the Heart Sound three to six times. Practice more to alleviate problems such as a sore throat, cold sores, swollen gums or tongue, jumpiness, moodiness, and heart disease.

5. Spleen: the Fifth Healing Sound

Associated organs: pancreas, stomach
Element: earth
Season: Indian summer

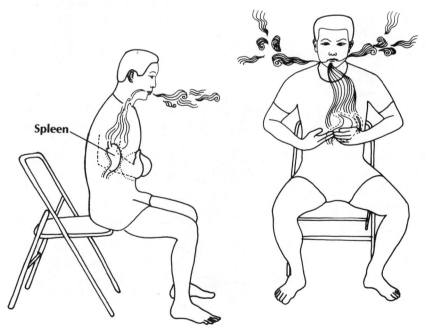

FIGURE APP. 1-10
The Spleen Sound
Place your hands with the three middle fingers resting at the bottom of the sternum, slightly to the left. Press in with the fingers

236

Color: yellow
Emotions: worry/fairness
Parts of the body: lips, mouth
Senses: taste
Taste: sweet, neutral
Sound: WHOOOOOO (from the throat, guttural)

a. Position: Take a deep breath as you place your hands beneath the sternum with the index fingers resting at the bottom rib, slightly to the left and above the navel. Press in with the fingers as you push out the middle back. (Figure App. 1-10)

b. Sound: Look up, and gently push your fingertips into the solar plexus area. Exhale the sound "WHOOOOOO" sub-vocally. Feel the sound vibrate the vocal cords. Feel your worries being expelled.

c. Rest and Concentrate: Once you have fully exhaled, close your eyes. Place your hands on your thighs, palms up, and concentrate your smiling energy on the spleen, pancreas, and stomach. Breathe into these organs. Imagine a bright yellow light shining, and feel the emotions associated with fairness growing.

d. Repeat the Spleen Sound three to six times. Practice more times to eliminate indigestion, nausea, and diarrhea.

6. Triple Warmer: the Sixth Healing Sound

The Triple Warmer refers to the three energy centers of the body: the upper section (brain, heart and lungs) is hot; the middle section (liver, kidneys, stomach, pancreas, and spleen) is warm; and the lower

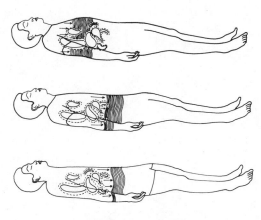

FIGURE APP. 1-11
The Triple Warmer

237

section (large and small intestines, bladder, and sexual organs) is cool. The Triple Warmer Sound, "HEEEEEEE," serves to balance the temperature between the three centers.

a. Position: Lie on your back with your arms resting at your sides, palms up, and your eyes closed. Inhale fully into all three cavities: chest, solar plexus, and lower abdomen.

b. Sound: Exhale the sound "HEEEEEEE" sub-vocally, first flattening your chest, then your solar plexus, and finally your lower abdomen. (Figure App. 1-11) Imagine a large roller pressing out your breath from your forehead to the pubic area.

c. Rest and Concentrate: When you have fully exhaled, concentrate on the entire digestive tract; that is, most of the torso.

d. Repeat the Triple Warmer Sound three to six times. Practice more to relieve insomnia (until you fall asleep) and stress.

APPENDIX 2:
DETAILED MERIDIAN POINTS

The following illustrations define each meridian by certain well-known acupuncture points. Most points are indicated by an abbreviation of the specific meridian and a number. (i.e., P-3 is point number 3 on the Pericardium Meridian.) There are two good books of reference outlining these points: *Acupuncture: A Comprehensive Text—The Shanghai College of Traditional Medicine*, translated and edited by John O'Conner and Dan Bensky, and *Anatomical Atlas of Chinese Acupuncture Points*, published by the Shandong Science and Technology Press.

The numbers are not always exactly the same for each point in both texts; therefore, the second label for a given point in this text is shown in parentheses. (This number represents the point indicated by the *Anatomical Atlas of Chinese Acupuncture Points*.) In addition you will find Chinese names labeling the more important points of this text in parentheses. YOU DO NOT NEED TO LEARN THE POINTS OF EACH MERIDIAN. You only need to know the lines associated with each meridian. The points are illustrated as guidelines and for informational purposes.

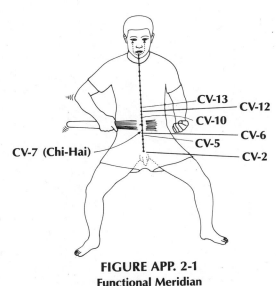

FIGURE APP. 2-1
Functional Meridian

239

1. Hit to awaken, detoxify, and strengthen the Lower Abdomen (Lower Tan Tien, or Chi Hai) (Figure App. 2-1)

2. Hit the Ming Men, or Door of Life, GV-4. (Figure App. 2-2)

3. Hit the Insides of the Elbows, P-3 (Quze.) (Figure App. 2-3)

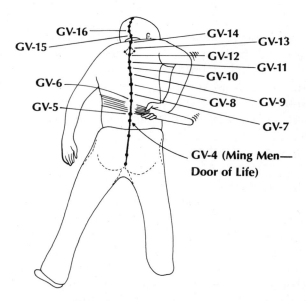

FIGURE APP. 2-2
Governor Channel

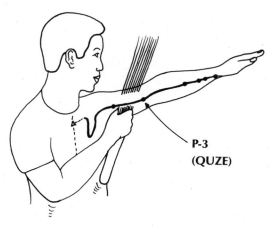

FIGURE APP. 2-3
Section of the Pericardium Meridian

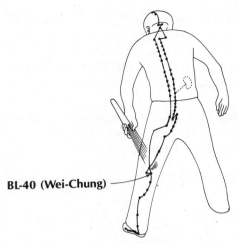

FIGURE APP. 2-4
The Urinary Bladder Meridian

BL-40 (Wei-Chung)

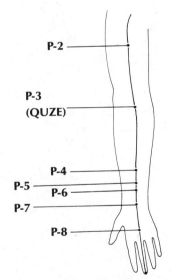

P-2

P-3
(QUZE)

P-4

P-5
P-6

P-7

P-8

FIGURE APP. 2-5
The Pericardium Meridian

4. Hit the Backs of the Knees, Bl-54 (BL40) (Wei Chung.) (Figure App. 2-4)

5. The Six Channels of the Left Arm and Hand:

a. Inside Elbow—Middle Finger Line—the Pericardium Meridian (Figure App. 2-5): Hit Point P-3 (Quze) three times. The specific points along the length of the meridian are hit as follows: P-2, P-3, P-4, P-5, P-6, P-7, wrist, P-8, palm, and middle finger.

 b. Inside Elbow—Thumb Line—the Lung Meridian (Figure App. 2-6): Hit Point LU-5 (Chize) three times. The route runs through the following points: LU-1, LU-2, LU-3, LU-4, LU-5, LU-6, LU-7, LU-8, LU-9, and LU-10.

 c. Inside Elbow—Pinkie Finger Line—the Heart Meridian (Figure App. 2-7): Hit Point H-3 (Shaohai) three times. The route runs as follows: H-1, H-2, H-3, H-4, H-5, H-6, H-7, and H-8.

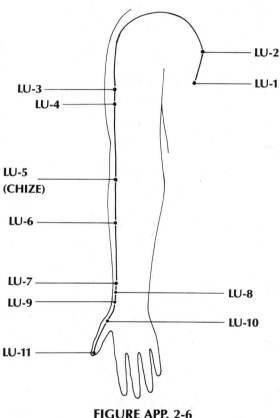

FIGURE APP. 2-6
The Lung Meridian

 d. Outside Elbow—Index Finger Line—the Large Intestine Meridian (Figure App. 2-8): Hit Point LI-5 (Quchi) three times. The points of the route are as follows: LI-15, LI-14, LI-13, LI-12, LI-11, LI-10, LI-9, LI-8, LI-7, LI-6, LI-5, and LI-4.

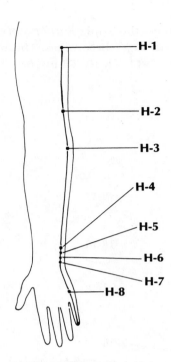

FIGURE APP. 2-7
The Heart Meridian

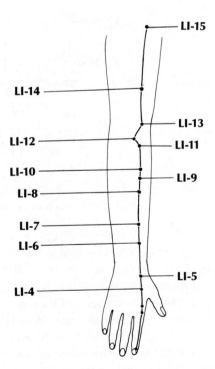

FIGURE APP. 2-8
The Large Intestine Meridian

e. Outside Elbow—Four Finger Line—the Triple Burner Meridian (Figure App. 2-9): Hit Point TB-10 (Tian Jing) three times. The route runs as follows: TB-14, TB-13, TB-12, TB-11, TB-10, TB-9, TB-8, TB-7, TB-6, TB-5, TB-4, and TB-3.

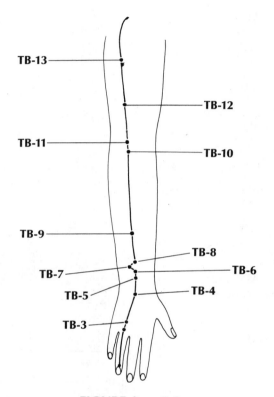

FIGURE App. 2-9
The Triple Burner (Warmer) Meridian

f. Outside Elbow—Pinkie Finger Line—the Small Intestine Meridian (Figure App. 2-10): Hit Point SI-8 (Xiao Hai) three times. The route runs as follows: SI-9, SI-8, SI-7, SI-6, SI-5, and SI-4.

6. The Six Meridians of the Leg

a. Back Side of Left Leg—Heel Line—the Bladder Meridian (Figure App. 2-11): The Bladder Meridian points are as follows: BL-54 (BL-40) (Wei Chung) (at the back of the knee), up to BL-49, BL-48, BL-47 (BL-52)(three inches to the left of the Door of Life). Hit back down the same line, returning to the back of the knee, and continue down to BL-55, BL-56, BL-57, BL-59, and BL-60.

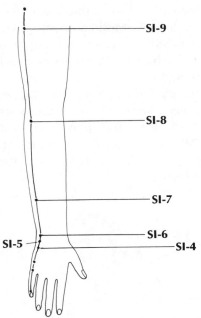

FIGURE APP. 2-10
The Small Intestine Meridian

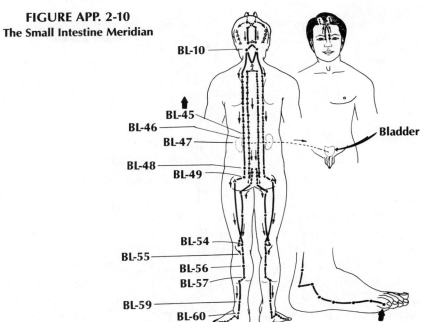

FIGURE APP. 2-11
The Urinary Bladder Meridian

245

b. Outside of the Left Leg—Fourth Toe Line—the Gall Bladder Meridian (Figure App. 2-12): The Gall Bladder Meridian points are as follows: GB-33 (Yang Kuan) (on the outside of the left knee), up to GB-32, GB-31, and GB-30 (Huan Tiao) (at the hip), and then back down to the knee, GB-34, GB-35, GB-36, GB-37, and GB-38.

c. Inside of Left Leg—Big Toe Line—the Spleen, Liver, Kidney Meridians (Figure App. 2-13): The Spleen Meridian points are as follows: SP-9 (Yin Ling Chuan), up to SP-10, SP-11, and then downward past SP-9 again, to SP-8, SP-7, and SP-6 (San Yin Chiao) (where the Spleen, Liver and Kidney Meridians meet). Hit SP-6 three extra times, then hit to the upper part of SP-5, and to the big toe.

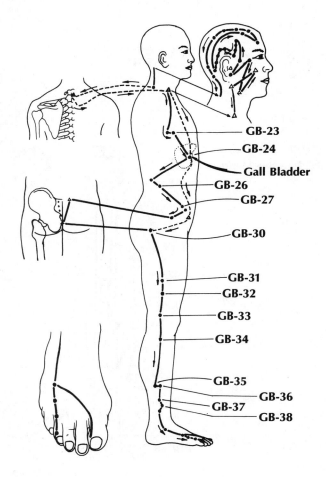

GB-23
GB-24
Gall Bladder
GB-26
GB-27
GB-30
GB-31
GB-32
GB-33
GB-34
GB-35
GB-36
GB-37
GB-38

FIGURE APP. 2-12
The Gall Bladder Meridian

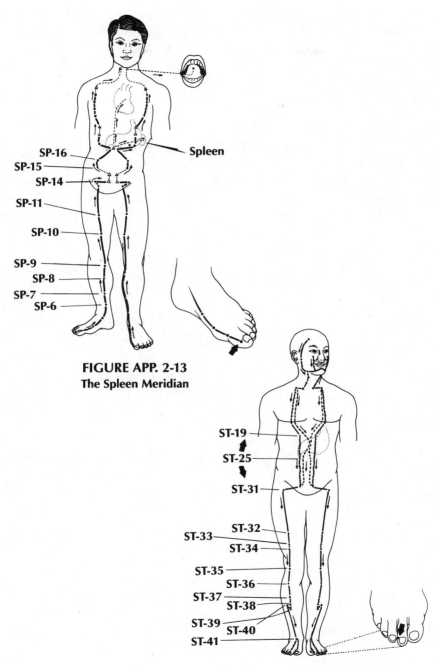

FIGURE APP. 2-13
The Spleen Meridian

FIGURE APP. 2-14
The Stomach Meridian

d. Front Side of Left Leg—Middle Toe Line—the Stomach Meridian (Figure App. 2-14): The Stomach Meridian points are as follows: ST-35 (Tu Pi) (under the kneecap), up to ST-34, ST-33, ST-32, ST-31, and back down the same route past the kneecap, to ST-36, ST-37, ST-38, ST-39, ST-40, and ST-41. Hit ST-41 three extra times. End the Hitting of this leg by Hitting Point BL-54 (BL-40) (Wei Chung) at the center of the inside of the knee.

7. The Meridians of the Back:

a. The Middle Line of the Back—the Governor Meridian (Figure App. 2-15): Hit GV-4 (the Ming Men Point, or Door of Life) three times. The points of the route are as follows: GV-6, GV-7, GV-8, GV-9, GV-10, GV-11, GV-12, GV-13, GV-14, GV-15 (Yamen), and GV-16 (Feng Fu). Gently hit this area an extra three times, then hit down to GV-2 (the sacrum).

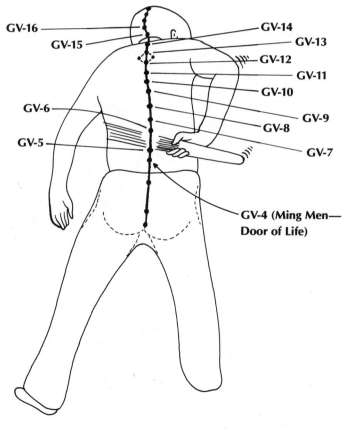

FIGURE APP. 2-15
The Governor Channel

b. The Left and Right Lines of the Back—the Bladder Meridian (Figure App. 2-16): Hit BL-47 (BL-52) (Zhishi) three times. The points of this route are as follows: BL-47 (BL-52), BL-46 (BL-51), BL-45 (BL-50), up to BL-10 and BL-9. Hit these points an extra three times, and down again past BL-47 (BL-52), down to BL-49 (BL-54) (at the side of the sacrum). Hit this point an extra three times. Then hit back up again to BL-47 (BL-52) (the Door of Life), hitting it an extra three times.

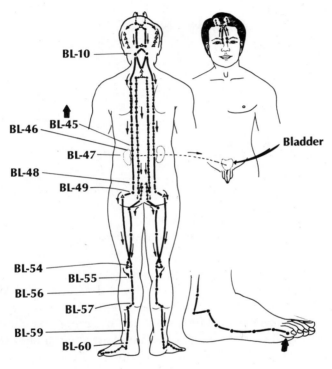

FIGURE APP. 2-16
The Urinary Bladder Meridian

8. The Front Part of the Body:

a. The Conception Vessel Meridian (Figure App. 2-17):

(1) Hit the Lower Tan Tien one and a half inches below the navel in men; three inches below the navel in women.

(2) The Conception Vessel Meridian—Above the Navel: Begin by Hitting Point CV-13, just below the xiphoid process. Hit downward to CV-12, midpoint between the xiphoid process and navel, and hit in a rolling fashion to CV-10, about an inch and a half above the navel.

249

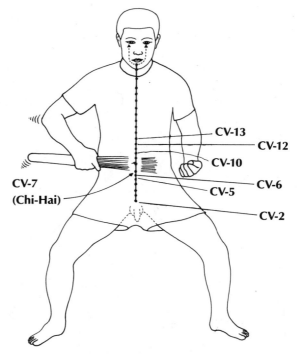

FIGURE APP. 2-17
The Conception Vessel Meridian

(3) Navel, Sexual Organs, Prostate/Ovaries of the Conception Vessel Meridian—the Middle Tan Tien: The Conception Vessel Meridian points below the navel are as follows: CV-8 (Chi Cgung) (the middle of the navel), down to CV-7, CV-6 (Chi Hai; one and a half inches below the navel—the Lower Tan Tien of men), down to CV-5, CV-4 (Kuan Yuan) (about three inches below the navel—the Lower Tan Tien of women), CV-3, CV-2, and back up to the navel.

b. Left Abdomen—the Stomach Meridian, one and a half inches to the left of the navel (Figure App. 2-18): The Stomach Meridian points are as follows: ST-25 (Tien Shu; one and a half inches to the left of the navel), down to ST-24, ST-23, ST-22, ST-21, ST-20, ST-19, up to just below the rib cage, and down to the left of the navel.

c. Left Abdomen—the Spleen Meridian, three inches to the left of the navel (Figure App. 2-19): The Spleen Meridian points are as follows: SP-15 (Ta Heng) (three inches to the left of the navel), downward to SP-14, SP-13, up the same line to SP-16 (below the rib cage), and back down to SP-15.

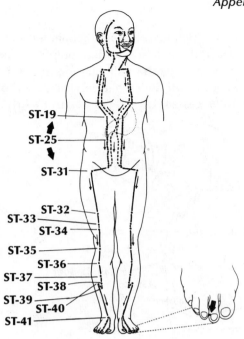

FIGURE APP. 2-18
The Stomach Meridian

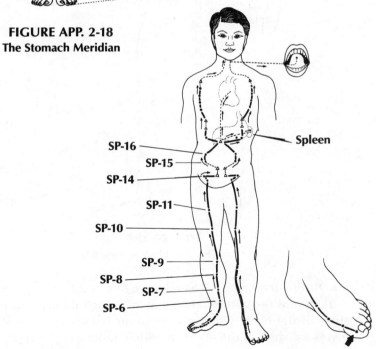

FIGURE APP. 2-19
The Spleen Meridian

d. Side of the Left Abdomen—the Gall Bladder Meridian far left side of the body (Figure App. 2-20): The Gall Bladder Meridian points are as follows: the GB-26 (Tai Mo), also known as the Belt Channel point, is very important in the development of the Belt Channel. Hit down to the left hip GB-27, and up GB-25, GB-24, GB-23, GB-22, and to the armpit.

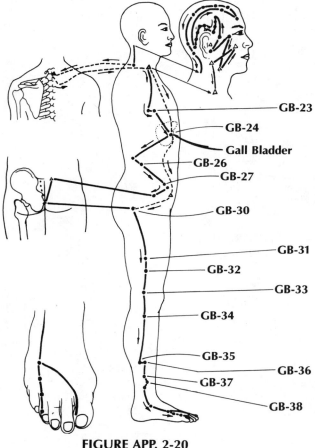

GB-23
GB-24
Gall Bladder
GB-26
GB-27
GB-30
GB-31
GB-32
GB-33
GB-34
GB-35
GB-36
GB-37
GB-38

FIGURE APP. 2-20
The Gall Bladder Meridian

e. Hitting the Left Rib Cage (Figure App. 2-21):

(1) Start at the bottom, right side of the left rib cage, directly at the center of the chest where the sternum is located. Hit following the downward angle of the rib the meridian points: KI-21, ST-19, and SP-16.

(2) Hit down the meridian line just below the nipple along the next rib beginning near the sternum the meridian points: KI-22, ST-18, and SP-17.

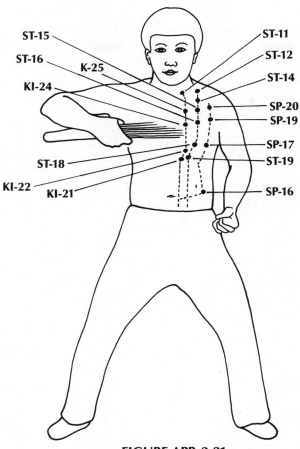

FIGURE APP. 2-21
The Points on the Left Rib Cage

(3) Hit down the meridian line just above the nipple, along the next higher rib, from the sternum down through the meridian points: KI-24, ST-16, and SP-19.

(4) Hit along the next higher rib, hitting from near the sternum downward, the meridian points: KI-25, ST-15, and SP-20.

(5) Hit downward along the next higher rib, just below the collarbone, beginning near the sternum, the meridian points: KI-26 and ST-14.

(6) Hit along the collarbone, starting from the top of the sternum and out toward the shoulder to the meridian points ST-11 and ST-12.

Bibliography

Alexander, Gerda. *Eutony*. Great Neck, New York: Felix Morrow, 1985.

Anatomical Atlas of Chinese Acupuncture Points. Jinan, China: Shandong Science and Technology Press, 1982.

Becker, Robert O. and Seldon, Gary. *The Body Electric: Electromagnetic Energy and the Foundations of Life*. New York: William Morrow and Company, Inc., 1985.

Chia, Mantak. *Awaken Healing Energy through the Tao*. New York: Aurora Press, 1983.

Chia, Mantak. *Chi Self-Massage: The Taoist Way of Rejuvenation*. New York: Healing Tao Books, 1986.

Chia, Mantak. *Healing Love through the Tao: Cultivating Female Sexual Energy*. New York: Healing Tao Books, 1986.

Chia, Mantak. *Iron Shirt Chi Kung I*. New York: Healing Tao Books, 1986.

Chia, Mantak. *Taoist Ways to Transform Stress into Vitality*.New York: Healing Tao Books, 1985.

Chia, Mantak, and Winn, Michael. *Taoist Secrets of Love: Cultivating Male Sexual Energy*. New York: Aurora Press, 1984.

Cousens, M.D., Gabriel. *Spiritual Nutrition and the Rainbow Diet*. Boulder, Colorado: Cassandra Press, 1986.

Grant, J.C. Boileau. *Grant's Atlas of Anatomy*. U.S.A.: The Williams and Wilkins Company, 1972.

Shanghai College of Traditional Medicine. *Acupuncture: A Comprehensive Text*, translated and edited by John O'Connor, and Dan Bensky. Chicago: Eastland Press, 1981.

Tart, Charles T. *The Open Mind*. El Cerrito, CA, 1986.

THE INTERNATIONAL HEALING TAO SYSTEM

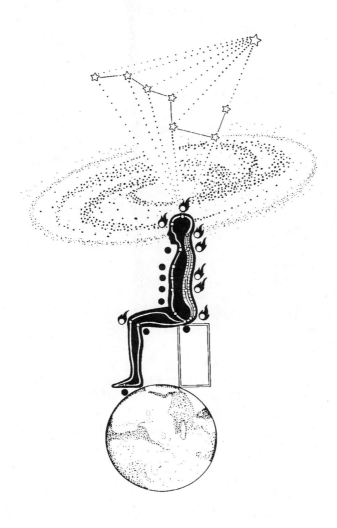

The Goal of the Taoist Practice

The Healing Tao is a practical system of self-development that enables the individual to complete the harmonious evolution of the physical, mental, and spiritual planes the achievement of spiritual independence.

Through a series of ancient Chinese meditative and internal energy exercises, the practitioner learns to increase physical energy, release tension, improve health, practice self-defense, and gain the ability to heal oneself and others. In the process of creating a solid foundation of health and well-being in the physical body, the basis for developing one's spiritual independence is also created. While learning to tap the natural energies of the Sun, Moon, Earth, and Stars, a level of awareness is attained in which a solid spiritual body is developed and nurtured.

The ultimate goal of the Tao practice is the transcendence of physical boundaries through the development of the soul and the spirit within man.

International Healing Tao Course Offerings

There are now many International Healing Tao centers in the United States, Canada, Bermuda, Germany, Netherlands, Switzerland, Austria, France, Spain, India, Japan, and Australia offering personal instruction in various practices including the Microcosmic Orbit, the Healing Love Meditation, Tai Chi Chi Kung, Iron Shirt Chi Kung, and the Fusion Meditations.

Healing Tao Warm Current Meditation, as these practices are also known, awakens, circulates, directs, and preserves the generative life-force called Chi through the major acupuncture meridians of the body. Dedicated practice of this ancient, esoteric system eliminates stress and nervous tension, massages the internal organs, and restores health to damaged tissues.

Outline of the Complete System of The Healing Tao

Courses are taught at our various centers. Direct all written inquiries to one central address or call:

The Healing Tao Center
c/o Order Fulfillment
400 Keystone Industrial Park
Dunmore, PA 18512
717-348-4310 - Fax 717-348-4313

INTRODUCTORY LEVEL I: Awaken Your Healing Light

Course 1: (1) Opening of the Microcosmic Channel; (2) The Inner Smile; (3) The Six Healing Sounds; and (4) Tao Rejuvenation—Chi Self-Massage.

INTRODUCTORY LEVEL II: Development of Internal Power

Course 2: Healing Love: Seminal and Ovarian Kung Fu.

Course 3: Iron Shirt Chi Kung; Organs Exercise and Preliminary Rooting Principle. The Iron Shirt practice is divided into three workshops: Iron Shirt I, II, and III.

Course 4: Fusion of the Five Elements, Cleansing and Purifying the Organs, and Opening of the Six Special Channels. The Fusion practice is divided into three workshops: Fusion I, II, and III.

Course 5: Tai Chi Chi Kung; the Foundation of Tai Chi Chuan. The Tai Chi practice is divided into seven workshops: (1) Original Thirteen Movements' Form (five directions, eight movements); (2) Fast Form of Discharging Energy; (3) Long Form (108 movements); (4) Tai Chi Sword; (5) Tai Chi Knife; (6) Tai Chi Short and Long Stick; (7) Self-Defense Applications and Mat Work.

Course 6: Taoist Five Element Nutrition; Taoist Healing Diet.

INTRODUCTORY LEVEL III: The Way of Radiant Health

Course 7: Healing Hands Kung Fu; Awaken the Healing Hand—Five Finger Kung Fu.

Course 8: Chi Nei Tsang; Organ Chi Transformation Massage. This practice is divided into three levels: Chi Nei Tsang I, II, and III.

Course 9: Space Dynamics; The Taoist Art of Energy Placement.

INTERMEDIATE LEVEL: Foundations of Spiritual Practice

Course 10:
Lesser Enlightenment Kan and Li: Opening of the Twelve Channels; Raising the Soul, and Developing the Energy Body.

Course 11: Greater Enlightenment Kan and Li: Raising the Spirit and Developing the Spiritual Body.

Course 12: Greatest Enlightenment: Educating the Spirit and the Soul; Space Travel.

ADVANCED LEVEL: The Immortal Tao (The Realm of Soul and Spirit)

Course 13: Sealing of the Five Senses.
Course 14: Congress of Heaven and Earth.
Course 15: Reunion of Heaven and Man.

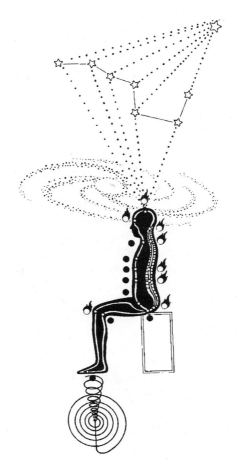

Course Descriptions of The Healing Tao System

INTRODUCTORY LEVEL I: Awaken Your Healing Light
Course 1:

A. The first level of the Healing Tao system involves opening the Microcosmic Orbit within yourself. An open Microcosmic Orbit enables you to expand outward to connect with the Universal, Cosmic Particle, and Earth Forces. Their combined forces are considered by Taoists as the Light of Warm Current Meditation.

Through unique relaxation and concentration techniques, this practice awakens, circulates, directs, and preserves the generative life-force, or Chi, through the first two major acupuncture channels (or meridians) of the body: the Functional Channel which runs down the chest, and the Governor Channel which ascends the middle of the back.

Dedicated practice of this ancient, esoteric method eliminates stress and nervous tension, massages the internal organs, restores health to damaged tissues, increases the consciousness of being alive, and establishes a sense of well-being. Master Chia and certified instructors will assist students in opening the Microcosmic Orbit by passing energy through their hands or eyes into the students' energy channels.

B. The Inner Smile is a powerful relaxation technique that utilizes the expanding energy of happiness as a language with which to communicate with the internal organs of the body. By learning to smile inwardly to the organs and glands, the whole body will feel loved and appreciated. Stress and tension will be counteracted, and the flow of Chi increased. One feels the energy descend down the entire length of the body like a waterfall. The Inner Smile will help the student to counteract stress, and help to direct and increase the flow of Chi.

C. The Six Healing Sounds is a basic relaxation technique utilizing simple arm movements and special sounds to produce a cooling effect

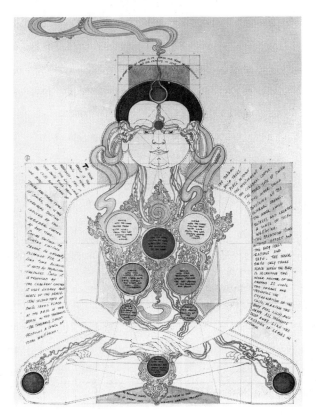

upon the internal organs. These special sounds vibrate specific organs, while the arm movements, combined with posture, guide heat and pressure out of the body. The results are improved digestion, reduced internal stress, reduced insomnia and headaches, and greater vitality as the Chi flow increases through the different organs.

The Six Healing Sounds method is beneficial to anyone practicing various forms of meditation, martial arts, or sports in which there is a tendency to build up excessive heat in the system.

D. Taoist Rejuvenation—Chi Self-Massage is a method of hands-on self-healing work using one's internal energy, or Chi, to strengthen and

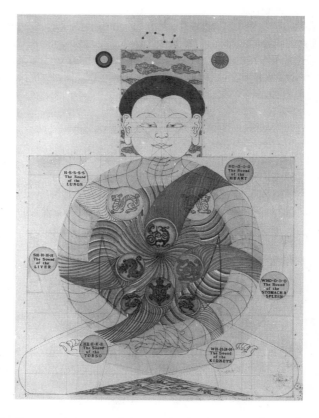

rejuvenate the sense organs (eyes, ears, nose, tongue), teeth, skin, and inner organs. Using internal power (Chi) and gentle external stimulation, this simple, yet highly effective, self-massage technique enables one to dissolve some of the energy blocks and stress points responsible for disease and the aging process. Taoist Rejuvenation dates back 5000 years to the Yellow Emperor's classic text on Taoist internal medicine.

Completion of the Microcosmic Orbit, the Inner Smile, the Six Healing Sounds, and Tao Rejuvenation techniques are prerequisites for any student who intends to study Introductory Level II of the Healing Tao practice.

INTRODUCTORY LEVEL II: Development of Internal Power

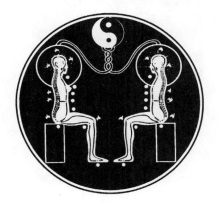

Course 2: *Healing Love: Seminal and Ovarian Kung Fu; Transforming Sexual Energy to Higher Centers, and the Art of Harmonious Relationships*

For more than five thousand years of Chinese history, the "no-outlet method" of retaining the seminal fluid during sexual union has remained a well-guarded secret. At first it was practiced exclusively by the Emperor and his innermost circle. Then, it passed from father to chosen son alone, excluding all female family members. Seminal and Ovarian Kung Fu practices teach men and women how to transform and circulate sexual energy through the Microcosmic Orbit. Rather than eliminating sexual intercourse, ancient Taoist yogis learned how to utilize sexual energy as a means of enhancing their internal practice.

The conservation and transformation of sexual energy during intercourse acts as a revitalizing factor in the physical and spiritual development of both men and women. The turning back and circulating of the generative force from the sexual organs to the higher energy centers of the body invigorates and rejuvenates all the vital functions. Mastering this practice produces a deep sense of respect for all forms of life.

In ordinary sexual union, the partners usually experience a type of orgasm which is limited to the genital area. Through special Taoist techniques, men and women learn to experience a total body orgasm without indiscriminate loss of vital energy. The conservation and transformation of sexual energy is essential for the work required in advanced Taoist practice.

Seminal and Ovarian Kung Fu is one of the five main branches of Taoist Esoteric Yoga.

Course 3:   *Iron Shirt Chi Kung;*
Organs Exercises and
Preliminary Rooting
Principle

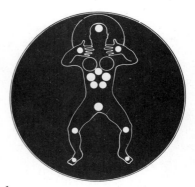

The Iron Shirt practice is divided into three parts: Iron Shirt I, II, and III.

The physical integrity of the body is sustained and protected through the accumulation and circulation of internal power (Chi) in the vital organs. The Chi energy that began to circulate freely through the Microcosmic Orbit and later the Fusion practices can be stored in the fasciae as well as in the vital organs. Fasciae are layers of connective tissues covering, supporting, or connecting the organs and muscles.

The purpose of storing Chi in the organs and muscles is to create a protective layer of interior power that enables the body to withstand unexpected injuries. Iron Shirt training roots the body to the Earth, strengthens the vital organs, changes the tendons, cleanses the bone marrow, and creates a reserve of pure Chi energy.

Iron Shirt Chi Kung is one of the foundations of spiritual practices since it provides a firm rooting for the ascension of the spirit body. The higher the spirit goes, the more solid its rooting to the Earth must be.

Iron Shirt Chi Kung I—Connective Tissues' and Organs' Exercise: On the first level of Iron Shirt, by using certain standing postures, muscle locks, and Iron Shirt Chi Kung breathing techniques, one learns how to draw and circulate energy from the ground. The standing postures teach how to connect the internal structure (bones, muscles, tendons, and fasciae) with the ground so that rooting power is developed. Through breathing techniques, internal power is directed to the organs, the twelve tendon channels, and the fasciae.

Over time, Iron Shirt strengthens the vital organs as well as the tendons, muscles, bones, and marrow. As the internal structure is strengthened through layers of Chi energy, the problems of poor posture and circulation of energy are corrected. The practitioner learns the importance of being physically and psychologically rooted in the Earth, a vital factor in the more advanced stages of Taoist practice.

Iron Shirt Chi Kung II—Tendons' Exercise: In the second level of Iron Shirt, one learns how to combine the mind, heart, bone structure, and Chi flow into one moving unit. The static forms learned in the first level of Iron Shirt evolve at this level into moving postures. The goal of Iron Shirt II is to develop rooting power and the ability to absorb and discharge energy through the tendons. A series of exercises allow the student to change, grow, and strengthen the tendons, to stimulate the vital organs, and to integrate the fasciae, tendons, bones, and muscles into one piece. The student also learns methods for releasing accumulated toxins in the muscles and joints of the body. Once energy flows freely through the organs, accumulated poisons can be discharged out of the body very efficiently without resorting to extreme fasts or special dietary aids.

Iron Shirt Chi Kung I is a prerequisite for this course.

Bone Marrow Nei Kung (Iron Shirt Chi Kung III)—Cleansing the Marrow: In the third level of Iron Shirt, one learns how to cleanse and

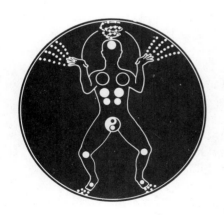

grow the bone marrow, regenerate sexual hormones and store them in the fasciae, tendons, and marrow, as well as how to direct the internal power to the higher energy centers.

This level of Iron Shirt works directly on the organs, bones, and tendons in order to strengthen the entire system beyond its ordinary capacity. An extremely efficient method of vibrating the internal organs allows the practitioner to shake toxic deposits out of the inner structure of each organ by enhancing Chi circulation. This once highly secret method of advanced Iron Shirt, also known as the Golden Bell System, draws the energy produced in the sexual organs into the higher energy centers to carry out advanced Taoist practices.

Iron Shirt Chi Kung is one of the five essential branches of Taoist Esoteric Practice.

Prior study of Iron Shirt Chi Kung I and Healing Love are prerequisites for this course.

Course 4: *Fusion of the Five Elements,*
Cleansing of the Organs, and
Opening of the Six Special Channels

Fusion of the Five Elements and Cleansing of the Organs I, II, and III is the second formula of the Taoist Yoga Meditation of Internal Alchemy. At this level, one learns how the five elements (Earth, Metal, Fire, Wood,

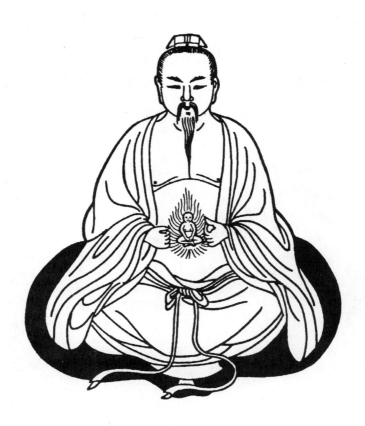

and Water), and their corresponding organs (spleen, lungs, heart, liver, and kidneys) interact with one another in three distinct ways: producing, combining, and strengthening. The Fusion practice combines the energies of the five elements and their corresponding emotions into one harmonious whole.

Fusion of the Five Elements I: In this practice of internal alchemy, the student learns to transform the negative emotions of worry, sadness, cruelty, anger, and fear into pure energy. This process is accomplished by identifying the source of the negative emotions within the five organs of the body. After the excessive energy of the emotions is filtered out of the organs, the state of psycho/physical balance is restored to the body. Freed of negative emotions, the pure energy of the five organs is crystallized into a radiant pearl or crystal ball. The pearl is circulated in the body and attracts to it energy from external sources—Universal Energy, Cosmic Particle Energy, and Earth Energy. The pearl plays a central role in the development and nourishment of the soul or energy body. The energy body then is nourished with the pure (virtue) energy of the five organs.

Fusion of the Five Elements II: The second level of Fusion practice teaches additional methods of circulating the pure energy of the five organs once they are freed of negative emotions. When the five organs are cleansed, the positive emotions of kindness, gentleness, respect, fairness, justice, and compassion rise as a natural expression of internal balance. The practitioner is able to monitor his state of balance by observing the quality of emotions arising spontaneously within.

The energy of the positive emotions is used to open the three channels running from the perineum, at the base of the sexual organs, to the top of the head. These channels collectively are known as the Thrusting Channels or Routes. In addition, a series of nine levels called the Belt Channel is opened, encircling the nine major energy centers of the body.

Fusion of Five Elements III: The third level of Fusion practice completes the cleansing of the energy channels in the body by opening the positive and negative leg and arm channels. The opening of the Microcosmic Orbit, the Thrusting Channels, the Belt Channel, the Great Regulator, and Great Bridge Channels makes the body extremely permeable to the circulation of vital energy. The unhindered circulation of energy is the foundation of perfect physical and emotional health.

The Fusion practice is one of the greatest achievements of the ancient Taoist masters, as it gives the individual a way of freeing the body of negative emotions, and, at the same time, allows the pure virtues to shine forth.

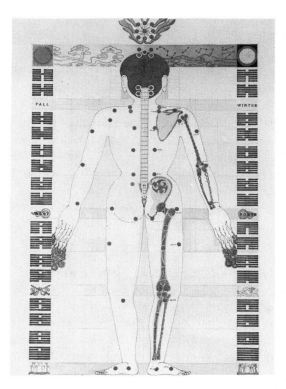

Course 5: *Tai Chi Chi Kung; The Foundation of Tai Chi Chuan*

The Tai Chi practice is divided into seven workshops: (1) the Original Thirteen Movements' Form (five directions, eight movements); (2) Fast Form of Discharging Energy; (3) Long Form (108 movements); (4) Tai Chi Sword; (5) Tai Chi Knife; (6) Tai Chi Short and Long Stick; (7) Self-Defense Applications and Mat Work.

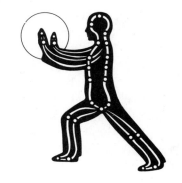

Through Tai Chi Chuan the practitioner learns to move the body in one unit, utilizing Chi energy rather than muscle power. Without the circulation of Chi through the channels, muscles, and tendons, the Tai Chi Chuan movements are only physical exercises with little effect on the inner structure of the body. In the practice of Tai Chi Chi Kung, the increased energy flow developed through the Microcosmic Orbit, Fusion work, and Iron Shirt practice is integrated into ordinary movement, so that the body learns more efficient ways of utilizing energy in motion. Improper body movements restrict energy flow causing energy blockages, poor posture, and, in some cases, serious illness. Quite often, back problems are the result of improper posture, accumulated tension, weakened bone structure, and psychological stress.

Through Tai Chi one learns how to use one's own mass as a power to work along with the force of gravity rather than against it. A result of increased body awareness through movement is an increased awareness of one's environment and the potentials it contains. The Tai Chi practitioner may utilize the integrated movements of the body as a means of self-defense in negative situations. Since Tai Chi is a gentle way of exercising and keeping the body fit, it can be practiced well into advanced age because the movements do not strain one's physical capacity as some aerobic exercises do.

Before beginning to study the Tai Chi Chuan form, the student must complete: (1) Opening of the Microcosmic Orbit, (2) Seminal and Ovarian Kung Fu, (3) Iron Shirt Chi Kung I, and (4) Tai Chi Chi Kung.

Tai Chi Chi Kung is divided into seven levels.

Tai Chi Chi Kung I is comprised of four parts:

a. Mind: (1) How to use one's own mass together with the force of gravity; (2) how to use the bone structure to move the whole body with very little muscular effort; and (3) how to learn and master the thirteen movements so that the mind can concentrate on directing the Chi energy.

b. Mind and Chi: Use the mind to direct the Chi flow.

c. Mind, Chi, and Earth force: How to integrate the three forces into one unit moving unimpeded through the bone structure.

d. Learn applications of Tai Chi for self-defense.

Tai Chi Chi Kung II—Fast Form of Discharging Energy:

a. Learn how to move fast in the five directions.

b. Learn how to move the entire body structure as one piece.

c. Discharge the energy from the Earth through the body structure.

Tai Chi Chi Kung III—Long Form Tai Chi Chuan:

a. Learn the 108 movements form.

b. Learn how to bring Chi into each movement.

c. Learn the second level of self-defense.

d. Grow "Chi eyes."

Tai Chi Chi Kung IV—the Tai Chi Sword.
Tai Chi Chi Kung V—Tai Chi Knife.
Tai Chi Chi Kung VI—Tai Chi Short and Long Stick.
Tai Chi Chi Kung VII—Application of Self-Defense and Mat Work.
Tai Chi Chuan is one of the five essential branches of the Taoist practice.

Course 6: *Taoist Five Element Nutrition; Taoist Healing Diet*
Proper diet in tune with one's body needs, and an awareness of the seasons and the climate we live in are integral parts of the Healing Tao. It is not enough to eat healthy foods free of chemical pollutants to have good health. One has to learn the proper combination of foods according to the five tastes and the five element theory. By knowing one's predominant element, one can learn how to counteract imbalances inherent in one's nature. Also, as the seasons change, dietary needs vary. One must know how to adjust them to fit one's level of activity. Proper diet can become an instrument for maintaining health and cultivating increased levels of awareness.

INTRODUCTORY LEVEL III: The Way of Radiant Health

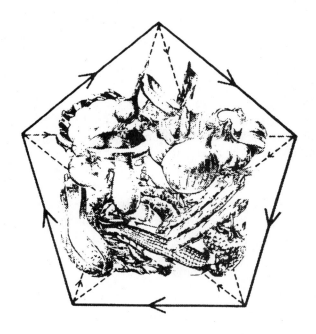

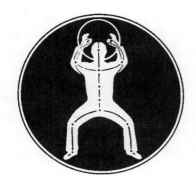

Course 7: *Healing Hands Kung Fu; Awaken the Healing Hand—Five Finger Kung Fu*

The ability to heal oneself and others is one of the five essential branches of the Healing Tao practice. Five Finger Kung Fu integrates both static and dynamic exercise forms in order to cultivate and nourish Chi which accumulates in the organs, penetrates the fasciae, tendons, and muscles, and is finally transferred out through the hands and fingers. Practitioners of body-centered therapies and various healing arts will benefit from this technique. Through the practice of Five Finger Kung Fu, you will learn how to expand your breathing capacity in order to further strengthen your internal organs, tone and stretch the lower back and abdominal muscles, regulate weight, and connect with Father Heaven and Mother Earth healing energy; and you will learn how to develop the ability to concentrate for self-healing.

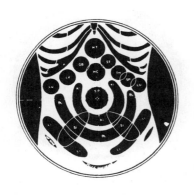

Course 8: *Chi Nei Tsang; Organ Chi Transformation Massage*

The practice is divided into three levels: Chi Nei Tsang I, II, and III.

Chi Nei Tsang, or Organ Chi Transformation Massage, is an entire system of Chinese deep healing that works with the energy flow of the five major systems in the body: the vascular system, the lymphatic system, the nervous system, the tendon/muscle system, and the acupuncture meridian system.

In the Chi Nei Tsang practice, one is able to increase energy flow to specific organs through massaging a series of points in the navel area. In Taoist practice, it is believed that all the Chi energy and the organs, glands, brain, and nervous system are joined in the navel; therefore, energy blockages in the navel area often manifest as symptoms in other parts of the body. The abdominal cavity contains the large intestine, small intestine, liver, gall bladder, stomach, spleen, pancreas, bladder, and sex organs, as well as many lymph nodes. The aorta and vena cava divide into two branches at the navel area, descending into the legs.

Chi Nei Tsang works on the energy blockages in the navel and then follows the energy into the other parts of the body. Chi Nei Tsang is a very deep science of healing brought to the United States by Master Mantak Chia.

Course 9: *Space Dynamics; The Taoist Art of Placement*

Feng Shui has been used by Chinese people and emperors for five thousand years. It combines ancient Chinese Geomancy, Taoist Metaphysics, dynamic Psychology, and modern Geomagnetics to diagnose energy, power, and phenomena in nature, people, and buildings. The student will gain greater awareness of his own present situation, and see more choices for freedom and growth through the interaction of the Five Elements.

INTERMEDIATE LEVEL: Foundations of Spiritual Practice

Course 10: *Lesser Enlightenment (Kan and Li); Opening of the Twelve Channels; Raising the Soul andDeveloping theEnergy Body*

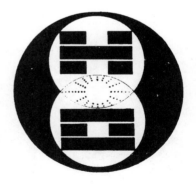

Lesser Enlightenment of Kan and Li (Yin and Yang Mixed): This formula is called *Siaow Kan Li* in Chinese, and involves a literal steaming of the sexual energy (Ching or creative) into life-force energy (Chi) in order to feed the soul or energy body. One might say that the transfer of the sexual energy power throughout the whole body and brain begins with the practice of Kan and Li. The crucial secret of this formula is to reverse the usual sites of Yin and Yang power, thereby provoking liberation of the sexual energy.

This formula includes the cultivation of the root (the Hui-Yin) and the heart center, and the transformation of sexual energy into pure Chi at the navel. This inversion places the heat of the bodily fire beneath the coolness of the bodily water. Unless this inversion takes place, the fire simply moves up and burns the body out. The water (the sexual fluid) has the tendency to flow downward and out. When it dries out, it is the end. This formula reverses normal wasting of energy by the highly advanced method of placing the water in a closed vessel (cauldron) in the body, and then cooking the sperm (sexual energy) with the fire beneath. If the water (sexual energy) is not sealed, it will flow directly into the fire and extinguish it or itself be consumed.

This formula preserves the integrity of both elements, thus allowing the steaming to go on for great periods of time. The essential formula is to never let the fire rise without having water to heat above it, and to never allow the water to spill into the fire. Thus, a warm, moist steam is produced containing tremendous energy and health benefits, to regrow all the glands, the nervous system, and the lymphatic system, and to increase pulsation.

The formula consists of:
1. Mixing the water (Yin) and fire (Yang), or male and female, to give birth to the soul;
2. Transforming the sexual power (creative force) into vital energy (Chi), gathering and purifying the Microcosmic outer alchemical agent;
3. Opening the twelve major channels;
4. Circulating the power in the solar orbit (cosmic orbit);
5. Turning back the flow of generative force to fortify the body and the brain, and restore it to its original condition before puberty;
6. Regrowing the thymus gland and lymphatic system;
7. Sublimation of the body and soul: self-intercourse. Giving birth to the immortal soul (energy body).

Course 11: *Greater Enlightenment (Kan and Li); Raising the Spirit and Developing the Spiritual Body*
This formula comprises the Taoist Dah Kan Li (Ta Kan Li) practice. It uses the same energy relationship of Yin and Yang inversion but increases to an extraordinary degree the amount of energy that may be

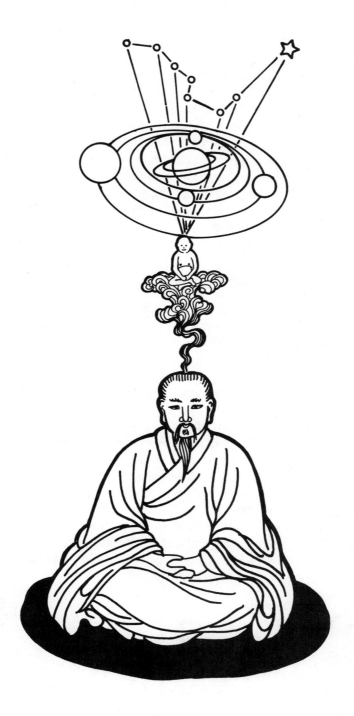

drawn up into the body. At this stage, the mixing, transforming, and harmonizing of energy takes place in the solar plexus. The increasing amplitude of power is due to the fact that the formula not only draws Yin and Yang energy from within the body, but also draws the power directly from Heaven and Earth or ground (Yang and Yin, respectively), and adds the elemental powers to those of one's own body. In fact, power can be drawn from any energy source, such as the Moon, wood, Earth, flowers, animals, light, etc.

The formula consists of:
1. Moving the stove and changing the cauldron;
2. Greater water and fire mixture (self-intercourse);
3. Greater transformation of sexual power into the higher level;
4. Gathering the outer and inner alchemical agents to restore the generative force and invigorate the brain;
5. Cultivating the body and soul;
6. Beginning the refining of the sexual power (generative force, vital force, Ching Chi);
7. Absorbing Mother Earth (Yin) power and Father Heaven (Yang) power. Mixing with sperm and ovary power (body), and soul;
8. Raising the soul;
9. Retaining the positive generative force (creative) force, and keeping it from draining away;
10. Gradually doing away with food, and depending on self sufficiency and universal energy;
11. Giving birth to the spirit, transferring good virtues and Chi energy channels into the spiritual body;
12. Practicing to overcome death;
13. Opening the crown;
14. Space travelling.

Course 12: *Greatest Enlightenment (Kan and Li)*

This formula is Yin and Yang power mixed at a higher energy center. It helps to reverse the aging process by re-establishing the thymus glands and increasing natural immunity. This means that healing energy is radiated from a more powerful point in the body, providing greater benefits to the physical and ethereal bodies.

The formula consists of:
1. Moving the stove and changing the cauldron to the higher center;
2. Absorbing the Solar and Lunar power;
3. Greatest mixing, transforming, steaming, and purifying of sexual

power (generative force), soul, Mother Earth, Father Heaven, Solar and Lunar power for gathering the Microcosmic inner alchemical agent;

4. Mixing the visual power with the vital power;
5. Mixing (sublimating) the body, soul and spirit.

ADVANCED LEVEL: The Immortal Tao
The Realm of Soul and Spirit
Course 13: *Sealing of the Five Senses*

This very high formula effects a literal transmutation of the warm current or Chi into mental energy or energy of the soul. To do this, we must seal the five senses, for each one is an open gate of energy loss. In other words, power flows out from each of the sense organs unless there is an esoteric sealing of these doors of energy movement. They must release energy only when specifically called upon to convey information.

Abuse of the senses leads to far more energy loss and degradation than people ordinarily realize. Examples of misuse of the senses are as follows: if you look too much, the seminal fluid is harmed; listen too much, and the mind is harmed; speak too much, and the salivary glands are harmed; cry too much, and the blood is harmed; have sexual intercourse too often, and the marrow is harmed, etc.

Each of the elements has a corresponding sense through which its elemental force may be gathered or spent. The eye corresponds to fire; the tongue to water; the left ear to metal; the right ear to wood; the nose to Earth.

The fifth formula consists of:

1. Sealing the five thieves: ears, eyes, nose, tongue, and body;
2. Controlling the heart, and seven emotions (pleasure, anger, sorrow, joy, love, hate, and desire);
3. Uniting and transmuting the inner alchemical agent into life-preserving true vitality;
4. Purifying the spirit;
5. Raising and educating the spirit; stopping the spirit from wandering outside in quest of sense data;
6. Eliminating decayed food, depending on the undecayed food, the universal energy is the True Breatharian.

Course 14: *Congress of Heaven and Earth*

This formula is difficult to describe in words. It involves the incarnation of a male and a female entity within the body of the adept. These two entities have sexual intercourse within the body. It involves the mixing of the Yin and Yang powers on and about the crown of the head, being totally open to receive energy from above, and the regrowth of the pineal gland to its fullest use. When the pineal gland has developed to its fullest potential, it will serve as a compass to tell us in which direction our aspirations can be found. Taoist Esotericism is a method of mastering the spirit, as described in Taoist Yoga. Without the body, the Tao cannot be attained, but with the body, truth can never be realized. The practitioner of Taoism should preserve his physical body with the same care as he would a precious diamond, because it can be used as a medium to achieve immortality. If, however, you do not abandon it when you reach your destination, you will not realize the truth.

This formula consists of:
1. Mingling (uniting) the body, soul, spirit, and the universe (cosmic orbit);
2. Fully developing the positive to eradicate the negative completely;
3. Returning the spirit to nothingness.

Course 15: *Reunion of Heaven and Man*

We compare the body to a ship, and the soul to the engine and propeller of a ship. This ship carries a very precious and very large diamond which it is assigned to transport to a very distant shore. If your ship is damaged (a sick and ill body), no matter how good the engine is, you are not going to get very far and may even sink. Thus, we advise against spiritual training unless all of the channels in the body have been properly opened, and have been made ready to receive the 10,000 or 100,000 volts of super power which will pour down into them. The Taoist approach, which has been passed down to us for over five thousand years, consists of many thousands of methods. The formulae and practices we describe in these books are based on such secret knowledge and the author's own experience during over twenty years of study and of successively teaching thousands of students.

The main goal of Taoists:
1. This level—overcoming reincarnation, and the fear of death through enlightenment;
2. Higher level—the immortal spirit and life after death;
3. Highest level—the immortal spirit in an immortal body. This body functions like a mobile home to the spirit and soul as it moves through the subtle planes, allowing greater power of manifestation.

Healing Tao Books

THE INNER STRUCTURE OF TAI CHI: Tai Chi Chi Kung I

This book is designed for Tai Chi practitioners of all levels. Stripping away the unnecessary mystery surrounding Tai Chi, Taoist Master Mantak Chia demonstrates, with the help of hundreds of drawings and detailed illustrations by Juan Li, the relationship of the inner structure of Tai Chi to the absorption, transformation, and circulation of the Three Forces, or energies —the Universal Force, the Cosmic Force, and the Earth 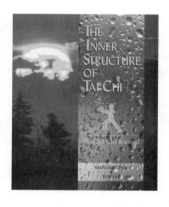 Force— that enliven us. The Inner Structure of Tai Chi is an indespensable resource for anyone who now practices or wants to learn a form of Tai Chi. Illustrated by Juan Li. Softbound. 182 pages.

$14.95 plus $3.95 for postage & handling
(Foreign Shipping: Please see page Catalog-38)
Order by Item No. B12

AWAKEN HEALING LIGHT *Of The Tao*

This book contains procedures that have been refined with over ten years of teaching experience at hundreds of workshops and feedback from thousands of students. *Awaken Healing Light of the Tao* clearly presents the most comprehensive instructions (basic and advanced) for realizing and developing our inherent energetic potentials. It explains in simple terms how to use the power of the mind to refine, transform, and 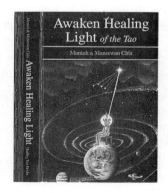 guide energy through the two primary acupuncture channels of the body which comprise the Microscomic Orbit. Practical methods for strengthening the immune system, recycling stressful energies, and restoring vibrant health are included. Illustrated by Juan Li. Softbound. 640 pages.

$16.95 plus $3.95 for postage & handling
(Foreign Shipping: Please see page Catalog-38)
Order by Item No. B11

TAOIST SECRETS OF LOVE: CULTIVATING MALE SEXUAL ENERGY

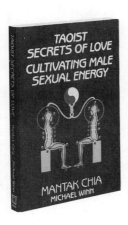

Master Mantak Chia reveals for the first time to the general public the ancient sexual secrets of the Taoist sages. These methods enable men to conserve and transform sexual energy through its circulation in the Microcosmic Orbit, invigorating and rejuvenating the body's vital functions. Hidden for centuries, these esoteric techniques make the process of linking sexual energy and transcendent states of consciousness accessible to the reader.

This revolutionary book teaches: Higher Taoist practices for alchemical transmutation of body, mind, and spirit; The secret of achieving and maintaining full sexual potency;

The Taoist "valley orgasm"—pathway to higher bliss;

How to conserve and store sperm in the body;

The exchange and balancing of male and female energies within the body, and with one's partner;

How this can fuel higher achievement in career, personal power, and sports.

This book, co-authored with Michael Winn, is written clearly, and illustrated with many detailed diagrams. Softbound. 250 pages.

$16.00 plus $3.95 for postage & handling
(Foreign Shipping: Please see page Catalog-38)
Order by Item No. B02

HEALING LOVE THROUGH THE TAO: CULTIVATING FEMALE SEXUAL ENERGY

This book outlines the methods for cultivating female sexual energy. Master Mantak Chia and Maneewan Chia introduce for the first time in the West the different techniques for transforming and circulating female sexual energy. The book teaches: The Taoist internal alchemical practices to nourish body, mind, and spirit;

How to eliminate energy loss through menstruation;

How to reduce the length of menstruations;

How to conserve and store ovary energy in the body;

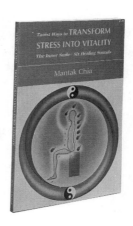

The exchange and balance of male and female energies within the body, and with one's partner;

How to rejuvenate the body and mind through vaginal exercises.

Written in clear language by Master Mantak Chia and Maneewan Chia. Published by Healing Tao Books. Softbound. 328 pages.

$14.95 plus $3.95 for postage & handling
(Foreign Shipping: Please see page Catalog-38)
Order by Item No. B06

TAOIST WAYS TO TRANSFORM STRESS INTO VITALITY

The foundations of success, personal power, health, and peak performance are created by knowing how to transform stress into vitality and power using the techniques of the Inner Smile and Six Healing Sounds, and circulating the smile energy in the Microcosmic Orbit.

The Inner Smile teaches you how to connect with your inner organs, fall in love with them, and smile to them, so that the emotions and stress can be transformed into creativity, learning, healing, and peak performance energy.

The Six Healing Sounds help to cool down the system, eliminate trapped energy, and clean the toxins out of the organs to establish organs that are in peak condition. By Master Mantak Chia. Published by Healing Tao Books. Softbound. 156 pages.

$10.95 plus $3.95 for postage & handling
(Foreign Shipping: Please see page Catalog-38)
Order by Item No. B03

CHI SELF-MASSAGE: THE TAOIST WAY OF REJU-VENATION

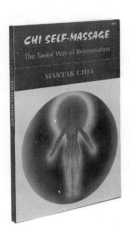

Tao Rejuvenation uses one's internal energy or Chi to strengthen and rejuvenate the sense organs (eyes, ears, nose, tongue), the teeth, the skin, and the inner organs. The techniques are five thousand years old, and, until now, were closely guarded secrets passed on from a Master to a small group of students, with each Master only knowing a small part. For the first time the entire system has been pieced together in a logical sequence, and is presented in such a way that only five or ten minutes of practice daily will improve complexion, vision, hearing, sinuses, gums, teeth, tongue, internal organs, and general stamina. (This form of massage is very different from muscular massage.)

By Master Mantak Chia. Published by Healing Tao Books. Softbound. 176 pages.

$10.95 plus $3.95 for postage & handling
(Foreign Shipping: Please see page Catalog-38)
Order by Item No. B04

IRON SHIRT CHI KUNG I: INTERNAL ORGANS EXERCISE

The main purpose of Iron Shirt is not for fighting, but to perfect the body, to win great health, to increase performance, to fight disease, to protect the vital organs from injuries, and to lay the groundwork for higher, spiritual work. Iron Shirt I teaches how to increase the performance of the organs during sports, speech, singing, and dancing.

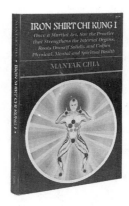

Learn how to increase the Chi pressure throughout the whole system by Iron Shirt Chi Kung breathing, to awaken and circulate internal energy (Chi), to transfer force through the bone structure and down to the ground. Learn how to direct the Earth's power through your bone structure, to direct the internal power to energize and strengthen the organs, and to energize and increase the Chi pressure in the fasciae (connective tissues).

By Master Mantak Chia. Published by Healing Tao Books. Softbound. 320 pages.

$14.95 plus $3.95 for postage & handling
(Foreign Shipping: Please see page Catalog-38)
Order by Item No. B05

BONE MARROW NEI KUNG: IRON SHIRT CHI KUNG III

Bone Marrow Nei Kung is a system to cultivate internal power. By absorbing cosmic energy into the bones, the bone marrow is revitalized, blood replenished, and the life-force within is nourished. These methods are known to make the body impervious to illness and disease. In ancient times, the "Steel Body" attained through this practice was a coveted asset in the fields of Chinese medicine and martial arts. Taoist methods of "regrowing" the bone marrow are crucial to rejuvenating the body, which in turn rejuvenates the mind and spirit. This system has not been revealed before, but in this ground-breaking work Master Chia divulges the step-by-step practice of his predecessors.

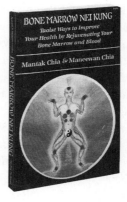

By Master Mantak Chia and Maneewan Chia. Published by Healing Tao Books. Softbound. 288 pages.

$14.95 plus $3.95 for postage & handling
(Foreign Shipping: Please see page Catalog-38)
Order by Item No. B08

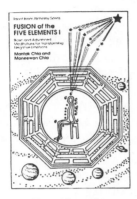

FUSION OF THE FIVE ELE-MENTS I

Fusion of the Five Elements I, first in the Taoist Inner Alchemy Series, offers basic and advanced meditations for transforming negative emotions. Based on the Taoist Five Element Theory regarding the five elemental forces of the universe, the student learns how to control negative energies and how to transform them into useful energy. The student also learns how to create a pearl of radiant energy and how to increase its power with additional internal energy (virtue energy) as well as external sources of energy—Universal, Cosmic Particle, and Earth. All combine in a balanced way to prepare the pearl for its use in the creation of an energy body. The creation of the energy body is the next major step in achieving the goal of creating an immortal spirit. Master Mantak Chia leads you, step by step, into becoming an emotionally balanced, controlled, and stronger individual as he offers you the key to a spiritual independence.

$12.95 plus $3.95 for postage & handling
(Foreign Shipping: Please see page Catalog-38)
Order by Item No. B09

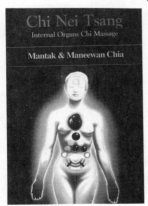

CHI NEI TSANG
(Internal Organ Chi Massage)

Chi Nei Tsang presents a whole new understanding and approach to healing with detailed explanations of self-healing techniques and methods of teaching others to heal themselves. Also included are ways to avoid absorbing negative, sick energies from others.

The navel's center is where negative emotions, stress, tension, and sickness accumulate and congest. When this occurs, all vital functions stagnate. Using Chi Nei Tsang techniques in and around the area of the navel provides the fastest method of healing and the most permanent results.

By Master Mantak Chia and Maneewan Chia. Published by Healing Tao Books. Softbound. 448 pages.

$16.95 plus $3.95 for postage & handling
(Foreign Shipping: Please see page Catalog-38)
Order by Item No. B10

AWAKEN HEALING ENERGY THROUGH THE TAO

Learn how to strengthen your internal organs and increase circulation through the flow of Chi energy. By Master Mantak Chia. Softbound. 193 pages.

$12.50 plus $3.95 for postage & handling
Order by Item No. B01

HEALING TAO INSTRUCTORS' BOOKS

LIVING IN THE TAO by THE PROFESSOR

This book is a Healing Tao instructor's accumulation of knowledge and wisdom from a volume of books and life experiences attained through his practice and instruction. An insider's view at life in the Tao.

- $9.95 plus $3.95 for postage & handling—**Order by Item No. IB01**

THE TAO AND THE TREE OF LIFE by Eric Yudelove

Using the basic structure of the Shamanic Universe, this book provides a context in which to examine the concepts, philosophy, and practical work of Taoist Internal Alchemy. Revealing parallels between Hebrew and western traditions, and long-lost sexual and alchemical secrets, hidden in the Zohar and Sepher Yetzirah.

- $14.95 plus $3.95 for postage & handling–**Order by Item No. IB02**

THE TAO OF NATURAL BREATHING by Dennis Lewis

- $17.95 plus $3.95 for postage & handling–**Order by Item No. IB03**

FORTHCOMING PUBLICATIONS

Cosmic Chi Kung—Techniques developing healing hands and ability to heal from a distance.

Five Element Nutrition—Ancient Chinese cooking based on the Five Elements Theory.

Fusion of the Five Elements II—Thrusting and Belt Channels. Growing positive emotions, psychic and emotional self-defense.

COSMIC COMIC BOOKS

Join us for some enlightened humor. Our first theme comic book—$5.95, add $3.95 for shipping and handling.

Item	Title
CB01	The Inner Smile (Energy Medicine of the Future)

VHS VIDEOS

Invite Master Chia into your living room.

Guided videos 30-60 minutes long $29.95 per tape. Please order by Item Number. Our videos are available in PAL System. **Add postage and handling as follows: 1 video—$3.95, 2 videos—$5.75, 3 or more videos—$6.50. (Foreign Shipping**: Please see page Catalog-38)

Item	Title
V40-G	Home Basic Sitting Meditation (complements V61)
V41-G	Home Basic Standing Meditation
V42-G	Inner Smile
V43-G	Six Healing Sounds

Workshop videos 60-120 minutes long, one tape $39.95; 2 tapes set $69.95 .

Item	Title
V50-TP	Tai Chi Chi Kung I (set of 2 tapes)
V51-TP	Tai Chi Chi Kung II (set of 2 tapes)
V52-TP	Chi Self Massage
V57-TP	Iron Shirt Chi Kung I
V58-TP	Iron Shirt III—Bone Marrow Nei Kung (2 tapes)
V59-TP	Iron Shirt II—Tendons exercises (set of 2 tapes)
V60-TP	Cosmic Chi Kung (Basic and Advanced Buddha Palm)

V61-TM Awaken Healing Light (set of 2 tapes)
V63-TP Healing Love through The Tao (set of 2 tapes)
V64-TM Fusion of Five Elements I (set of 2 tapes)
V65-TM Fusion of Five Elements II (set of 2 tapes)
V66-TM Fusion of Five Elements III (set of 2 tapes)
V67-TP Chi Nei Tsang (set of 2 tapes)
V68-P Chi Nei Tsang's Healing Power Practice
V69-TP Tao-In: Regaining a Youthful Body (set of 2 tapes)

CASSETTE TAPES

Guided Practice Tapes C09-C18 are guided by Master Mantak Chia.
$9.95 each, add $3.95 for shipping and handling.
(**Foreign Shipping**: Please see page Catalog-38)

Item	Title
C09	Inner Smile
C10	Six Healing Sounds
C11	Microcosmic Orbit
C11a	Healing Love
C12	Tai Chi Chi Kung I
C13	Iron Shirt Chi Kung I
C14	Sitting Meditation for Home Instruction
C15	Standing Meditation for Home Instruction
C16	Fusion of the Five Elements I
C17	Fusion of the Five Elements II
C18	Fusion of the Five Elements III

BONE MARROW NEI KUNG (IRON SHIRT III) EQUIPMENT

Only sold as listed!

Item No.	Title	Price	Postage & Handling
62C	Untreated Drilled Jade Egg	$15.95	$3.95
62DG	Chi Weight-Lifting Bar and Silk Cloth	25.95	7.25
62EF	Wire Hitter, Rattan Hitter, Bag for Equipment	39.95	7.25

CARDS

◆Eight Immortal Greeting cards sold in sets of 2 (16 cards in all). Full color, depicting the Eight Immortals with a short history of each one. Ideal for sharing with family and friends! **$9.95 per set.**
◆ Instructional formulas Chi Cards. Now also available in French.**$9.95 each.**
Add $3.95 for shipping and handling.

Item	Title
GC01	Eight Immortal Greeting Cards Set
CC01	Chi Cards - Level 1 (20 cards/set)
CC02	Chi Cards - Level 2 (18 cards/set)
CC03	Chi Cards - Level 3 (18 cards/set)

THE INTERNATIONAL HEALING TAO CENTERS:

AMERICA
- *BERMUDA*
- *CANADA*

Ontario
British Columbia
Quebec
- *UNITED STATES*

Alabama
Arizona
California
   Los Angeles
   San Francisco
Colorado
Connecticut
Delaware
Florida
Hawaii
Illinois

Kansas
Massachusetts
Michigan
Minnesota
New Hampshire
New Jersey
New Mexico
NewYork
North Carolina
Oklahoma
Oregon
Pennsylvania
South Dakota
Virginia

ASIA
- *INDIA*
- *JAPAN*

- *THAILAND*

AUSTRALIA

EUROPE
- *AUSTRIA*
- *ENGLAND*
- *FRANCE*
- *GREECE*
- *HOLLAND*
- *SWITZER-LAND*
- *NETHER-LANDS*
- *SPAIN*
- *GERMANY*
- *ITALY*

Our new center in Thailand holds retreats during the winter and summer seasons, and is located in Chiang Mai. For more information, please call, fax, or write to: The Healing Tao Center
274 Moo 7, Laung Nua
Doi Saket, Chiang Mai 50220
Phone: (66, 53) 495-596 through 599—Fax: (66, 53) 495-852

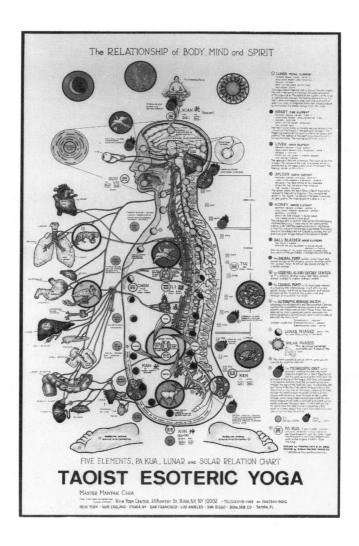

BODY/MIND/SPIRIT CHART 23" x 35", full-color chart by Susan McKay.
$7.50 per copy plus $3.95 for postage and handling
(Foreign Shipping: Please see page Catalog-38)
Order by Item No. C H47

POSTERS

18 x 22", four-color process posters were created by artist Juan Li. Please order by item number.

Sold as Poster set of 12 for $59.95
(Foreign Shipping: Please see page Catalog-38)
Order by Item No. 45.

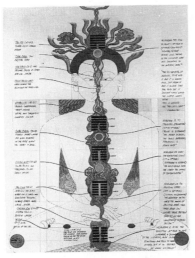

The Microcosmic Orbit—Small Heavenly Cycle—The Functional Channel (Yin). The Microcosmic Orbit Meditation is the key to circulating internal healing energy, and is the gateway to higher Taoist Meditations.
Item No. P31

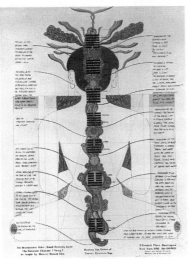

The Microcosmic Orbit—Small Heavenly Cycle—The Governor Channel (Yang). The Governor Channel of the Microcosmic Orbit Meditation allows the Yang (hot) energy to flow from the base of the spine to the brain.
Item No. P32

Healing Love and Sex—Seminal Kung Fu. By conserving their seeds during lovemaking, men can transform sexual energy into spiritual love, and, at the same time, enjoy a higher orgasm. The main purpose of Seminal and Ovarian Kung Fu is to utilize sexual energy for attaining higher levels of consciousness so that the sexual urge does not control the person.
Item No. P35

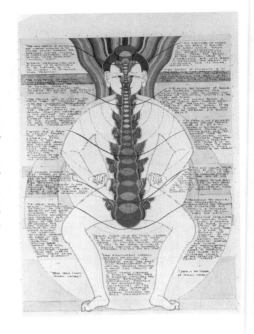

Healing Love and Sex—Ovarian Kung Fu. The Taoists teach women to regulate their menstrual flow and transmute sexual orgasm into higher spiritual love. The techniques of Seminal and Ovarian Kung Fu allow the practitioner to harness sexual impulses so that sex does not control the person. By controlling sexual impulses, people are able to move from the mortal level into higher levels of consciousness.
Item No. P36

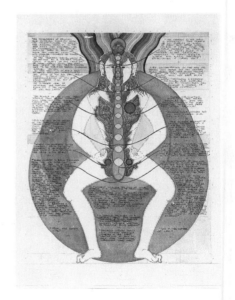

Fusion of the Five Elements I—Cleansing, Clearing, and Harmonizing of the Organs and the Emotions. Each organ stores a separate emotional energy. When fused into a single balanced Chi at the navel, the opening of the six special channels becomes possible.
Item No. P37

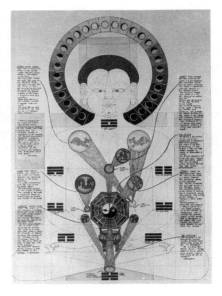

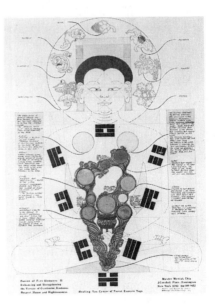

Fusion of the Five Elements II—Enhancing and Strengthening the Virtues. Fusion of the Five Elements II strengthens positive emotions, balances the organs, and encourages in men and women the natural virtues of gentleness, kindness, respect, honor, and righteousness.
Item No. P38

Fusion of the Five Elements II—Thrusting Channels. Running through the center of the body, the Thrusting Routes allow the absorption of cosmic energies for greater radiance and power.
Item No. P39

Fusion of the Five Elements II—Nine Belt Channel. The Taoist Belt Channel spins a web of Chi around the major energy vortexes in the body, protecting the psyche by connecting the power of Heaven and Earth. **Item No. P40**

The Harmony of Yin and Yang. "Yin cannot function without the help of Yang; Yang cannot function without the help of Yin." —Taoist Canon, 8th century A.D. **Item No. P41**

Pa Kua. The Cauldron of Fusing the Energy and Emotions. *Also sold separately, $7.50 each copy, add $3.95 for shipping and handling.*
Item No. P42➤

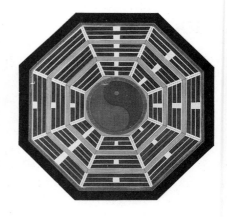

Fusion of the Five Elements III—Yin Bridge and Regulator Channels. Fusion of the Five Elements III uses special meridians to cleanse the aura and regulate high-voltage energy absorbed by the body during meditation. **Item No. P43**

Fusion of the Five Elements III—Yang Bridge and Regulator Channels. Fusion of the Five Elements III teaches the yogic secrets of safely regulating the release of the kundalini power using special meridians. **Item No. P44**

NEW PRODUCTS

POSTERS
$9.50 each add $3.95 shipping and handling.

The Inner Alchemy of the Tao. Beautifully illustrated chart. Instructional pamphlet is included. Item No. CH48

The Eight Immortal Forces. The legendary figures of the Eight Immortals are depicted in this chart with full explanations of their mysteries. Instructional pamphlet is included. **Item No. CH49**

BOOKS

THE MULTI-ORGASMIC MAN

In this book co-written by Master Mantak Chia and Doug Arava, and published by Harper Collins, you'll learn the amazing facts about the multi-orgasmic capabilities of men. By learning to separate orgasm and ejaculation—two distinct physical processes—men can transform a momentary release into countless peaks of whole body orgasms without losing an erection. In addition to becoming better sexual partners, multi-orgasmic men enjoy increased vitality and longetivity because they minimize the fatigue and depletion that follow ejaculation.

$20 plus $3.95 for postage & handling
(Foreign Shipping: Please see page Catalog-38)
Order by Item No. B13
Harper Collins Publisher
ISBN# 0-06-251335-4

HOW TO ORDER

Prices and Taxes:
Subject to change without notice. New York State residents please add 8.25% sales tax.

Payment:
Send personal check, money order, certified check, or bank cashier's check
to: THE HEALING TAO CENTER
          c/o Order Fulfillment
          400 Keystone Industrial Park
          Dunmore, PA 18512
          Tel. (717) 348 -4310 — FAX: (717) 348-4313

 All foreign checks must be drawn on a U.S. bank. Mastercard, Visa, and American Express cards accepted.

Shipping

Domestic Shipping: via UPS, requires a complete street address.   Allow 3-4 weeks for delivery.

Foreign Shipping: *European countries only: Worldmail by DHL, surface mail ($7.95 per book), air mail ($15.95 per book).* Courier service by air, as an alternative for traceable shipments or heavy orders, is also available as a collect service. For other products please see chart below.

Order Total	Domestic Zone 1-6	Domestic Zones 7 & 8	Foreign by Surface	Foreign by Air
$20.00 or less	$ 3.95	$ 3.95	$ 7.95	$15.95
20.01 - 40.00	6.95	7.25	17.95	30.95
40.01 - 60.00	8.50	9.25	27.50	45.95
60.01 - 80.00	9.75	10.75	37.95	60.95
80.01 - 100.00	11.00	12.75	47.95	75.95
100.01 - 120.00	12.25	14.50	57.95	90.95
120.01 - 140.00	13.50	16.25	67.95	105.95
140.01 - 200.00	16.50	21.50	97.95	150.95
Over 200.00	add $4.95/every$50		add $20.95 /every $50	add $40.95 /every $50

Zones 7 & 8—Zip codes with the first 3 digits:
577, 586 - 593, 677 - 679, 690, 693
733, 739, 763 - 772, 774 - 774, 778 - 797, 798 - 799
800 - 899, 900 - 994
All other Zip codes are Zones 1 - 6

❖**Please call or write for additional information in your area**❖